7/23/13

To Diann,

Thank you for the awareness and care you give to me, health needs always and that of my family. May these stories of wonderful woman inspire and touch your heart. In the darkness they look for Hope!

Sorority of Hope

Vicki

Small Cell Cervical Cancer and Large Cell Cervical Cancer Sisterhood

SCCC/LCCC

Melanie Cummins
Toni Petoskey
Vicki R. Reding

Copyright © 2012 Small Cell Cervical Cancer and Large Cell cervical Cancer Sisterhood

All rights reserved.

ISBN:1481991043
ISBN-13:978-1481991049

Small and Large Cell Neuroendocrine Carcinoma of the Uterine Cervix; Also known as Small or Large Cell Cervical Cancer (SCCC/LCCC), are rare and aggressive cancers. They are fast growing and spread rapidly. There is no known link to HPV and usually cannot be detected by a regular PAP screening. The prognosis is poor and there is no set protocol for treatment. Thank you for supporting the women of the SCCC/LCCC Sisterhood.

Proceeds from the sale of this book directly contribute to a SCCC/LCCC Research fund that is administered By MD Anderson Cancer Hospital in Texas. Our sisterhood has raised over $215,000 to date.

DEDICATION

JOURNEY: A DEDICATION TO THE WOMEN OF THIS SISTERHOOD BY VICKI L. REDING

Our life's journey takes us along many paths. Some are planned, others unexpected and then those moments so abrupt, they change everything in an instant.

Where do you turn when you have something so rare? You feel so very alone and as if no one else can understand or care.

From all over the world, a small group of women found their way home to one another. No two stories are the same. They, however, are stitched together by a thread that has formed this circle – this sisterhood.

These amazing women are not defined by their rare disease, but by the dedication, compassion and understanding they have found for one another.

They choose to encourage, uplift, support and offer a safe place to gather. To shoulder each other's burdens, vent frustrations and share their grief.

Remaining mindful to live each day with purpose and a grateful heart. Accepting joy when given and embracing laughter where found. Most of all to continue to be examples of HOPE…

The determination to find sunshine while weathering the storm inspires. Warriors in this battle, your strength astounds. The dignity, grace and love you have shown are a lesson in living well to all. You have made this world a better place. Wishing each of you PEACE…

This book is dedicated to all the sisters we have lost and all the sisters who will come.

Sorority of Hope

Introduction

In our darkest hour as humans, it can sometimes feel as if there will never be light again, or that the weight of our situation will never be lifted. Yet, somehow, the human spirit continues to overcome. We find a way. That is our nature. Hope is an everlasting gift we receive in life. As long as you keep hope close to your heart, there is always a tomorrow and it will lead you to that proverbial "light at the end of the tunnel".

Sometimes we seek out others in our own situation, for many different reasons. There is definitely hope when others come together and join those just starting a particular journey, and lead them by the hand, down the path they have just walked. To be able to lift people up in their time of need, when they are scared and unsure, and show them the promise of what might be, can lift your own spirit as well. No one should ever have to go through these trials alone.

When the SCCC/LCCC (Small Cell and Large Cell Cervical Cancer) Sisterhood was started, all that the founding members knew was that something special was happening. The women initiating the group had struggled through their own rare cancer diagnoses alone and terrified. Once the first two women found each other, they vowed no other woman would ever be alone in this fight. The movement took off and morphed into more than they had ever imagined. What they had thought would be a place to come and find comfort and support, became a place for resources, advice, inspiration and friendship. Until this group was formed, this type of resource did not exist for SCCC/LCCC. Without all of the women who have joined the group along the way, there would be no group as it stands today, making medical history, pioneering the use of Social Media in the new way the group has inspired. There would still be so many women struggling all alone and searching for answers.

"Sorority of Hope" is just what its name suggests. It is a sisterhood bound by the diagnosis of a terrible disease, yet an inspiring place of hope and faith with women from all walks of life and every corner of the world. Although most may never meet in person, the virtual relationships formed are more real and even stronger than most "real world" friendships. The group goes beyond your everyday "cancer support group" as each woman lifts up another to a height only understood by those in the sisterhood.

Hope is the main factor in this faction and it is the tie that binds. For without hope, you have nothing. Our sisterhood has everything!

Chapter 1

Imagine a day you hear the words "you have cancer". Some of you have already lived that day. Any cancer diagnosis is devastating and there is no "good" or "bad" cancer. But for others, who have never faced this diagnosis, imagine that the cancer with which you have been diagnosed is rare and aggressive. You are told the prognosis is poor, to say the least, and even warned not to research this type of cancer on the Internet. What little you find will scare the Hell out of you. You have questions, but get no real answers. Why is that? Because there are no real answers. Your options are all a guessing game and, although your doctors are knowledgeable, most have never dealt with a case like yours. The others have had nothing but bad outcomes when dealing with this cancer. A good doctor will give you hope and is willing to fight with you as long as you are able. Because the diagnosis of any cancer is grim, he will try to ease the blow in any way he can, without being untruthful. What a difficult job. Then....wait for it.....the odds are against you surviving more than 18 months past the date of diagnosis. Can you imagine that?

How many of you are women in your 20s or 30s with young children? How many of you reading this right now, may be a little older, married to the love of your life and have beautiful grandchildren? How many of you are 19, just married and have given birth to your first child, only to leave that baby motherless in just a few short months? How many of you live in a foreign country where this disease has never been seen, and the all-important screenings used to stay one step ahead of the cancer is not covered by insurance, and won't be provided? These women are all a part of our SCCC/LCCC "sisterhood".

Neuroendocrine Small Cell of the Uterine Cervix, also known as Small Cell Cervical cancer (SCCC), is a rare and aggressive cancer comprising about 1% of all cervical cancers diagnosed in the world each year. Because this cancer is so rare, there is no set protocol for treatment and the prognosis for survival is grim. Most women diagnosed are not given a lot of answers up front. They want and need more information, so they go searching. Most turn to the World Wide Web for answers and sadly there aren't many. What is found is crippling. Large Cell Cervical Cancer is much like SCCC, but thought possibly to be even more rare and differentiated by the size of the cell. Because of this, the Sisterhood has welcomed, with open arms, women with this diagnosis as well. There are a handful of sisters that have been diagnosed with these rare cancers originating in other areas of the pelvic region. This diagnosis is just as uncommon, if not more. They have also been welcomed into our group, as they have nowhere else to turn. No women should ever be alone in this fight. Because of this notion, the first step in the journey of this wonderful sisterhood was born and the rest is history.

Although the two women who initiated this movement found each other on a cancer message board, they did so because of one woman. She was truly the first SCCC/LCCC "sister", even though she passed more than a year before the group officially started. Here is her story, told by her sister and one of the supporters of our sisterhood today:

Meredith's story, written by Kerri Wright Stauffer

I was living in TN and my younger sister was living in North Bend, WA, a small town outside of Seattle. We were close. We talked a lot on the phone. I missed her terribly! She had just returned from London, spending the holidays with her fiancé. She had called me one evening and said, "I have something to tell you." I knew before she even said it. She was getting married. I was so happy for her. Little did we know that her world was about to be turned upside-down.

It was March 6th, 2005. My phone rang. It was my mother. I could tell something was wrong and she said Meredith asked her to get me on the phone. My heart sank. Meredith told me that she had some breakthrough bleeding that day and had Mom take her to the ER. After an exam, the ER doctor told her that he thought she had cervical cancer and needed to make an appointment with her gynecologist as soon as possible.

I could not believe what I was hearing. My first thought and response to Meredith was that the ER doctor should never tell someone they have cancer without a biopsy. The little I knew at the time about cervical cancer was that it was slow growing. I told Meredith it was ok. She would be fine. I really didn't think she had cervical cancer. I was looking for wanted reassurance.

The next day my mother got her in to see the gynecologist and he walked into the room saying, "These ER doctors diagnosing without a biopsy...." He did the pap and he told Meredith he was taking a few biopsies, and then left the room. He came back 10 minutes later and said he also believed it to be cervical cancer. He stated she had a mass on her cervix. He also made an appointment for her to see the gynecological oncologist the same week. He sent them straight over to the hospital to get a CAT scan. Meredith fell apart, scared beyond words. When they arrived at the hospital Meredith told my mother she couldn't get out of the car, she couldn't do it. My mother was at her strongest right at that moment. I could not imagine the fear she was feeling as well. She took Meredith's hand and said, "You don't have to think about anything. Your father and I will do that for you. All you have to do is put one foot in front of the other." Needless to say, she couldn't have the scan that day. She was so sick to her stomach, she could not hold down the contrast dye. I got a call that night and it devastated me. So all we knew was there was a tumor on the cervix and Meredith had another appointment with an oncologist the next Wed. I had so many thoughts running through my head. How in the world is my healthy, younger sister being told she has cancer? I could not wrap my head around this.

March 9th, 2005. The day the words, "Small Cell Cervical Cancer" came into my family's life. I was waiting for the call from Meredith. It came about 4:30 in the afternoon and when I picked up...she was laughing. I thought for that instant it was all a mistake. My sister is fine. I asked her what happened. She said it is not good. She had an aggressive type of cervical cancer and she was a stage IIIb. I could not believe what I was hearing. My younger sister: the picture of health and cancer in the same sentence. This wasn't happening.

I asked a few more questions and she told me the name of her cancer. The next words out of her mouth were, "Do not look it up, Kerri. The prognosis is bad." What?!?!?!? She said she starts chemo the next week. I was sitting there, 2,000 miles away from my sister, and she had cancer. WHY? I fell apart.

That night I spent all night reading about this cancer. Everything I could find on SCCC is that is has a poor prognosis and it is rare. There just wasn't anything out there about it.

Over the next week I told her I was moving to WA in the beginning of April. That would give me time to take care of work and get my son ready to move and so on. She was so depressed. Her fiancé flew in from London the minute he heard. Of course Mom, Dad and Alison were right there for her.

They noticed Meredith was not keeping any food down. My family just thought it was nerves. They did her blood work on Friday the 11th, and called my mom that Monday and said, "Get Meredith to the hospital at once." She was in kidney failure.

Now, in a week's time, my healthy sister was diagnosed with cancer and now in kidney failure. The tumor was so large it was causing her kidneys to back up and raise her creatine levels. She was rushed in for emergency surgery on Monday evening to put in 2 stints.

I got the call Tuesday morning from my other sister, Alison, about Meredith's condition. I said I am on my way. I put my son in the car Weds morning, the 16th of March, and drove to Seattle, WA. We arrived Saturday night. I knew Meredith had received her first round of chemo the day before, so I went to the hospital Sunday morning. I had not seen Meredith in about 9 months, maybe longer (her last visit to TN.) I walked in and her long, beautiful hair was cut short. I just hugged her and did not want to let her go. My mother was there. Meredith said she wanted McDonalds. We were all over that. She wanted to walk. Now Meredith was on the

11th floor. I DID NOT do elevators. I told my mom while Meredith was in the bathroom I was going to start walking down and would meet them in the lobby. She grabbed my arm and pulled me out in the hallway and said, "If your little sister can fight cancer, you can get on that elevator." I did.

I wasn't there right after Meredith had the kidney surgery, but I was told that they put her chemo off until her kidneys were functioning better. My sister sat in the hospital for 3 days begging them to give her chemo. The little she knew about Small Cell was it was fast growing and it responded well to chemo.

My mother said that they did not give her anything for nausea after her first round to see how she did with the chemo. It was horrible. Meredith ended up so violently sick that night. They had to carry her back to bed.

This was Meredith's 1st treatment, in her words, "I had Cisplatin and Etoposide, six rounds, five straight days, every three weeks. When I went in for the hysterectomy, they found residual tumor on the small intestine. Then I had more chemo, Cisplatin and Irinotecan once a week for four weeks, but they had to stop because the neuropathy got so bad. I also had roughly six weeks of external radiation and two internal radiation treatments. I was scheduled for four of those, but it was stopped because they could find no evidence of tumor on the cervix."

Around August, Meredith went in for her radical hysterectomy. I knew my family was going to be there and she would be in surgery most of the day. When I arrived I could not find my family in the waiting room. I asked at the desk for the Wright Family and she directed me to a quiet room. This is never a good sign. I walked in and could see my family had been crying. Everyone looked to be in a state of shock. I started to cry immediately. I thought we had lost Meredith during the surgery. My dad walked over and explained that they found residual cancer cells on her small intestines and her prognosis was very bad. I just could not believe this. All that treatment she just went through.

We went upstairs to see Meredith and we tried to put on happy faces. When she was wheeled in, she was very tired. She woke up and we were all sitting around her. She saw us and said, "What now?" My mother took her hand and explained what they had found, and that they were not able to finish the surgery. Meredith said, "Well that sucks! What do we do now?" She was ready to fight some more. She wasn't giving up. My mother wasn't about to let her oncologist give up either. My mother walked out into the hall and talked to Meredith's doctor and said, "What's the plan?" The doctor said she didn't have one. My mother very sternly said, "You will come up with a plan B!"

My mother was informed by the doctor, who had assisted Meredith's doctor in surgery that when the residual cells were found, and all the doctor could do was close Meredith, she cried. She knew she could not do anymore.

Now, on to the second oncologist, who I cannot say enough good things about. He was fantastic and Meredith really liked Dr. Goodman. He had experience with small cell cancer. He started another treatment and then great news. She went into remission in January 2006, for 10 wonderful months.

Through all her treatments, Meredith searched for anyone that had this cancer. She could not find anyone. She felt so alone. She found a website called Cancer Compass and there were just a couple of people on there with SCCC. Even through all her treatment she still found time to go onto Cancer Compass and try to help anyone that was going through this. Meredith was like that. She always tried to help other people before herself.

When it came time for the scans, we would sit on pins and needles. Then, in Oct 2006, her scan showed a hot spot. The cancer was back. Meredith started another round of chemo and a different type of radiation called Cyber Knife. This went on for some time.

I can't even begin to tell you what a fighter she was. She wanted to live. I remember a conversation I had with my Dad. Meredith would not be able to sleep and go into Dad's room and have long conversations. One conversation that, to this day, is hard for me. Meredith said she wasn't afraid to die, she was afraid that we will go on without her. I never understood that. How could she think that we would be able to move past losing her? I don't feel you ever move past losing a sister. It follows you every day of your life.

On Thanksgiving 2007, I cooked and Meredith was pretty sick by this time. I knew when she didn't take that last round of chemo that she wasn't taking anymore. She keep telling my mother when she feels better she will take it. But I knew better.

I took a plate up to Meredith that night and she nibbled on a green bean just to make me happy. She said she was tired and wanted some privacy. She was in my mother's room, at this point, and my mother slept on the couch next to the bed. My mother never left her side. I could tell Meredith was tired, so I walked over and gave her a hug and told her I *loved her. She said, "I love you, too." Those were the last words Meredith ever said to me.*

The next morning we were getting a Christmas tree and Mom called. She said Meredith was talking funny. Alison and I went straight over and by the time we got there, nothing was wrong. Meredith was talking fine. Mom said she called her heating pad a birthday cake. But she seemed fine. We were listening through the door. We didn't want Meredith to think mom was freaking out by calling us. So I went on with my husband and got a tree, took it home and put it up.

That evening I was sitting on my bed painting my toenails. I stopped and looked at Jason and said, "I have to go to Mom's right now. Something is wrong." I have no idea where that came from. We went to Mother's and Meredith was upstairs sleeping. Nothing was wrong. I still had this feeling that I needed to stay.

Our other sister, Heather, who was 2,000 miles away in TN, was up and cooking breakfast at 6 am, which made it 4 am our time. Heather had an overwhelming urge to call Mom. She had no idea why. She did not want to call, knowing she would wake Meredith. The feeling would not go away. So Heather called, and of course, it woke our mother. Heather didn't know what to say besides she had to call and let everyone know how much she missed them. That phone call woke my mother and she found Meredith in dire need of medical attention.

I had fallen asleep and my dad woke me at 4:30 am and said, "We have called an ambulance to take Meredith to the hospital." I jumped up and ran in there. Meredith was on the bed and you could tell she was in pain, just staring and breathing hard. I will never forget her face. I begged for God to help her.

Meredith never said anything. We got her to the hospital and the doctors were wonderful. They started pain meds the minute she came through the door. They took her down for a CAT scan because her stomach was hard. Everyone went but me. I had to call our other sister in TN and tell her what was going on. When I came back into the ER room they were still gone. There was a curtain between us and an older gentleman. I heard this loud nurse come in on his side and he said, "Shhhh! Don't you know there is a young girl next to me dying of cancer?" I broke. I wanted the doctors to fix whatever was wrong so my sister could come home.

They got her back to the ER and we waited. We were told they were trying to get her on the oncology floor and someone would be down to move her soon. We waited and waited. I finally walked out and looked at that doctor and said, "Please, please do not let my sister die in this emergency room." He said if he had to move her himself, it would be done. Just a few minutes later they moved her. We were in a private room. It was my younger sister Alison, Mom, Dad and I. Meredith was unresponsive all day. We talked to her though and we told stories about her and things we all had done together.

Meredith had a dog named, Ed. He was her baby. Ed was at the house and I knew Meredith would be upset if nobody was taking care of him. I also knew I could not watch my little sister take her last breath. I walked into the hallway and told my dad that. He said, "You have to do what is right for you in this time." I walked back into her room knowing this would be the last time I got to hold my sister. I *hugged her so tight and smelled her hair, rubbed her fingers in my hand and leaned into her ear and told her how very blessed I was to have her as my sister and that I loved her so much. I know she heard me. I have to believe that. I turned to walk out and ran back to her because I knew this was the last time. I didn't want to let her go. My husband was driving me to my mother's and my heart and soul were broken. They are still broken today, without her.*

My younger sister showed up at my mother's house just a little while after we arrived, and said she was getting a few things to go back and take up to the hospital. I was laying on Meredith's bed just crying, taking in her smell. Alison and I were sitting there talking and we had our other sister in TN on the phone. As we were talking, her phone rang. It was my dad telling us Meredith was gone. I just screamed her name out loud. I will never forget that feeling. You feel as if your soul has been ripped apart.

Meredith left us on Saturday, November 24, 2007, at 7:17 pm.

If Meredith were still here, she would fight to keep women informed about cervical cancer awareness and prevention. She is not here to do that, so I do it for her.

Meredith was asked by Dr. Goodman to write a paper for Swedish Hospital about her experience with Small Cell Cervical Cancer. This was Meredith's last paragraph. "Cancer is a bad hand to get dealt and difficult in so many ways- physically, mentally and spiritually – but one thing I think I can say with some confidence is that cancer has made me stronger."

Not a day goes by in my life that I do not miss my little

sister. I will for the rest of my life. If you have a sister, you know how very special they are.

Ladies, please get your PAPS and yearly well-woman checkups. Tell your mothers, aunts, cousins, friends, daughters, and your sisters. This doesn't have to be your story. I wish every day it wasn't mine.

Meredith....I love you

My name is Colleen Marlett, and when I was diagnosed with Neuroendocrine Small Cell of the Cervix, I did not know of Meredith or what her story and her passion to reach out to others would mean for me. I was diagnosed on August 14th, 2006. We had just bought the home of our dreams and we were living on the Central Coast of California, in the town where I grew up. It is a beautiful place and it was a beautiful time of year. This diagnosis was about to change everything.

I did the same as most of the other women and looked it up on the Internet. I had gone to the doctor on the 11th with a discharge. I had no other symptoms up until then. But looking back, I was very fatigued for about 10 months before the diagnosis. I had my regular PAP (that I never missed) in October of 2005, and everything was normal, as it had always been. By the end of the day on the 11th, I had seen a gynecologist who had done a biopsy. She wouldn't confirm what I already knew...it was cervical cancer. I could tell it was cancer by the look on everyone's faces. And it had to be cervical cancer because all she would tell me for sure, until the biopsy came back, was that there was an ugly looking "something" covering my cervix. She had never seen anything like it before.

I Googled cervical cancer the minute I got home. But everything I read talked about it being slow-growing and able to be detected, before becoming invasive, by a regular PAP (Papanicolaou Gynecological Smear Test). As I said, I never missed a one. I had a medical family history of breast cancer on my biological mother's side of the family. All the women older than I, but one, had not survived. I had Ductal Carcinoma In Situ in 2001. This is a non-invasive form of Breast Cancer, and I felt lucky (if there is such a thing with cancer). I told no one about the DCIS, except my mom. The others in my life knew only that I had a benign tumor and I was having it removed. I pushed it out of my head and went on with my life until I was stopped dead in my tracks with this secondary cancer, SCCC.

The more I read about the symptoms of cervical cancer the more I started to think this was something else... possibly uterine or ovarian cancer? Oh no. Please, no! Cervical Cancer was pretty treatable, but the symptoms didn't fit. Somewhere along the way, in my searching the Internet, something popped up about varying types of rare cervical cancers. Somewhere amongst those articles, I came across the words Small Cell Cervical Cancer. No! Monday, it was confirmed. I had cervical cancer. But, what type of cervical cancer? I asked how it could have grown so fast and the doctor had no answer. I asked for the pathology report and, without dragging this story along, after reading the report myself, I came to the conclusion this was, in fact, Small Cell. After trying to convince two doctors this was not your garden-variety cervical cancer, it was my radiologist who finally listened to my plea to take a closer look. He did. Three days later it was confirmed. This was Neuroendocrine Small Cell Cervical Cancer.

I Googled, again and again, but there was nothing. Only a snip-it here or there, stating this was rare and had a very poor prognosis and high probability for death within 6 to 18 months from diagnosis. My oncologist was much more optimistic, as well as my radiation oncologist. If I could get rid of this through the first treatments, I had an 80% chance of keeping it gone for good. But I had only a small chance of getting rid of it through treatment. I did not have surgery first, as they do know this type of tumor responds well to chemo with radiation, but spreads quickly if given any downtime. I went through the same treatment as Meredith did the first time, (chemo types and radiation types) and in April of 2007, I was cancer-free. I breathed a sigh of relief and now faced PET scans (Positron Emission Tomography), to make sure the cancer stayed gone, every three months for the unforeseeable future, living life one PET scan at a time.

In the interim of all this, my insurance did not cover much (another long story on how I ended up with the crap end of the deal for insurance), and with the lack of my income and all the medical expenses, our family suffered financial disaster (of which we are now just coming out of, 6 years later). Truth be told, that was my main focus through it all. My family was suffering a double whammy, all because I got sick. I could see the changes in my family, especially in my children. My husband just kept working and plugging along. We were split apart in different directions and I was at a loss to fix it. Once I was cancer free, it fell on me to handle the financial mess (which all I could really do was worry and keep us out of Bankruptcy) and deal with my silent fear that this cancer would come back. If it did, the doctors had already warned me they could not cure me at that point; they would only be able to prolong my life and make me comfortable.

The harsh treatments associated with the type of chemo and amount of radiation I had left me relatively unscathed at first. I will say I noticed a marked decline in my memory, eyesight and hearing, but all in all, I was in good shape. The weight had started to pour on, but the lack of energy and emotional eating I had taken to were overpowering. I was suffering emotionally, but silently. I was scared to death that this cancer would come back. However, I was never really afraid this cancer would take my life. Strange? I kept on moving forward, trying to keep the pieces of our lives together. But admittedly, looking back, I fell short. I felt so alone and isolated. There was no one I could talk to. The people who loved me wanted this all to be in the past and really couldn't relate to any of my fears or feelings of seclusion. I talked to other survivors of other cancers and found it made me feel even worse. Many uninformed people would say things like, "Why didn't you just have a hysterectomy and be done with it?" As if I wanted to go through all the pain and suffering I had. They didn't understand this wasn't the cervical cancer you hear about. Even the normal type of invasive cervical cancer will require more than a hysterectomy. I found that most people associated Cervical Cancer with what is actually the pre-cancerous stage, that can be taken care of with different options other than chemo and radiation. This diagnosis isn't actually cancer (yet), but people don't understand; even some of those in the medical profession don't get it. Worse yet, EVERYONE I talked to related Cervical Cancer to HPV. They made comments, either directly to me or to people I know, alluding to the fact they thought I got this because of a sexually transmitted disease, when in fact, I did not have

HPV. I had been screened several months before when the vaccination campaign was in full swing. In addition, and this is important information for all to understand, there was no HPV in the DNA of the tumor. This is one facet used to determine the type of cancer at biopsy. So, let me make this clear, Small Cell Cervical Cancer has no known link to HPV. Even if it did, did I deserve this potential death sentence? Does anyone who is diagnosed with HPV? Some women will have HPV, but the tumor will not. Neuroendocrine Small Cell Carcinoma is a common, yet very aggressive disease in the liver, lung and brain. What makes it so rare is the fact that it originated in the cervix. That is the difference. So I now say, "I had Small Cell that happened to originate in the cervix. Not cervical cancer; Two very different animals."

When I was first diagnosed and Googling everything, I did come across a cancer message board with a few women posting about having SCCC. The most prominent person posting was Meredith, from the story before. She was in remission and I remember getting a sense from her postings that she was reaching out to women with this diagnosis, in an effort to keep them informed by sharing her experiences and answering their fearful posts. I wasn't ready to be included in that crowd, so I read through the messages and then never went back to the Internet again...until after I had been cancer free for more than a year.

It was now May of 2008, and I had just had another "cancer free" PET scan. My worry of a recurrence started to lift a little, but the loneliness was getting the better of me. "What was the name of that message board?" I Googled again, this time resisting the urge to open the one or two articles that mentioned how deadly SCCC was and combing through for the message board only. I found it! It took a minute to sink in. No one had posted in some time. I scrolled back a few pages and this is what I found:

"What stage were you? I am so glad to hear you are doing so well!!!! I am Meredith's sister. You can see some of her post on here. We lost her on Nov. 24th*, 2007. I cannot tell you how it breaks my heart for her not to be here, but I know she would be so happy for you!*

Take care-

Kerri"

I was shocked. I never expected this. I was sure Meredith would be there. She seemed so full of life and she was so young. But she was gone. Oh no! My second thought, and the only real thought I have had on the subject since then, was, "Who would continue to reach out?" Kerri was doing a great job carrying on, but somehow Meredith's words of encouragement are what rang through my head. If she could make it, so could I. Without realizing it, I had clung to hope from the words of Meredith. I went back and read all the posts again. In almost every one of Meredith's posts, she ended with how she wished there was more information on this cancer and hoped all women could get the advice and support they needed. I had no intentions of adding my two cents to this group that day, but I was compelled in a split second to post to the group, hoping my words might reach someone, anyone in need. I wrote:

"By Collemarle on Tue May 06, 2008 05:00 PM

Hi, I am here and cancer free. I was diagnosed with Small Cell Cervical in August 2006. Stage 2b. I was 10 months from my last pap, which had been clear. I didn't have HPV.

The info I could find had all the women having hysterectomies with very little survival rate. I didn't have one. I had 7 rounds of chemo (whatever I could handle) and during the course I also did 35 days of external radiation and then 4 treatments of internal radiation. It took almost 7 months. I just zapped it the best I could!

They told me my prognosis was bleak. If I could get rid of the tumor completely the first time around my chances would be better of surviving 6 to 18 months.

I just went for my last PET CT in April of 2008, and I am still cancer free, now 13 months. No signs; none in my lungs, liver or brain. I have to say that my doctors are much more optimistic since it has been more than a year and the small cell has not returned anywhere else in the body.

I hope this message finds all the women battling this rare form of CC healthy and well. I read through this message board and I want everyone to know that just because they say you may not be able to beat this, they are wrong. They told me my chances were "slim to none". I never ever believed them. I still don't, even if it returns. I'll beat it. So can you. I want to put this behind me as well and the way I did that was to write a book. It was published on the same day as my one-year PET CT. You have no expiration date. That's between you and God. He put these scientists here for us. Use them wisely."

There were some posts from newly diagnosed patients that would later stop as they got into treatment or remission. There were still replies from Kerri and another woman named Mona, who would both later become one of our "sisters" and "sister supporters" as well, but for the most part, that was it. On August 6th, 2008, I was going through the message board and there was a posting from a woman who had been diagnosed in May of 2007, and was cancer free as well. She wrote:

"*Small Cell Cervical Cancer*

by cmel32 on Tue Aug 05, 2008 08:00 PM

Hi I am 44 years old, diagnosed with small cell cervical cancer May 1, 2007. I am looking for people living with this rare cancer to communicate with. It is very easy to feel alone when dealing with something so rare. I am 15 months post diagnosis and 1 year post treatment, with no signs of cancer. Melanie"

I don't know what struck me about her post, but just like the split second decision to post the last time, I made the same quick decision to reply to this woman, privately. With my fingers crossed for a friendly response from her, I wrote:

"Hi Melanie,

My name is Colleen and I am in the same boat as you. I am 2 years from diagnosis and cancer free almost 17 months now. Can you tell me a little about yourself?

How are you coping? Are you married? Kids? What part of the country are you from? Your age? I am starved to talk to someone in my same situation! As you have probably figured out, there aren't many of us.

I come from a long line of woman with one female cancer or another. I had breast cancer in 2001, and that was a walk in the park compared to this. I was 38 when I was diagnosed with SCCC. As you have probably figured out, not many of us survive this cancer, let alone actually ever be cancer free for more than 6 months after treatment. But, looks like we both have done that. I don't mean to sound like a downer, actually the opposite. Hurray!!!! We have already beaten the odds. People don't really understand just how bad this type of cancer is unless they are faced with it. Not to say that all cancer isn't horrible. It is. But not as many are like this, where not much is known. And it seems to me that not many people care about this cancer. It is hard to do on your own. I knew my chances were slim to get this far, cancer free, and I did it. Now I know, no matter what happens from one PET to the next, I will prevail.

I am happy to hear from you. I hope we can stay in touch.

Colleen Marlett"

The very next day I received this:

"Hi Colleen,

I am so happy to hear from you. I too feel like I am alone with this cancer. I don't even search the computer for information because it just freaks me out too badly.

I was diagnosed May 01, 2007, with stage 2b. I am single. Never been married and have never had any children. I live in Michigan, about 1 hour from Detroit. I have had a very hard time coping with all this. I am 44 years old. I feel like I have no one to talk to. Family and loved ones really can't handle all the thoughts that go through your mind. My biggest fear is that this may kill me. I feel also like no one understands what we are going through. I did not think I would still be here 1 year later as well. I am so very grateful, but still live with the fear of what the future holds.

I've worked at Henry Ford Hospital in Detroit, as an

Ultrasound Tech for the past 8 years. I recently had, in July, a PET scan that was clear. I do believe I have done better than they could have ever imagined when I started this journey. What did you do for treatment? I did chemo and internal and external radiation. Boy, no one could have prepared me for the internal radiation. I was very lucky to have a great radiation oncologist. He was my saving grace. He just moved to Chicago and I told him that's ok, I will do my visits there. The thought of getting a new doctor makes me want to scream, so off to Chicago I go in September for my visit. I go to gyne oncologist every 4 months. Do you still see your radiation doctor? How often do you see your oncologist?

I also would like to hear about your life. I have had a lot of cancer in my family. I lost my father June 2004, to lung cancer, and since my diagnosis, I've lost both his sisters to cancer - one to leukemia and one to skin cancer. I also feel starved to talk to someone in my situation. I hope we can keep in close touch and get to know each other and be there for each other. I do believe it will help us both to have someone to talk to. We are going to be the ones that beat this.

Thank you for writing. I look forward to hearing from you.

Melanie Cummings"

For the next couple of days we exchanged emails. They were long and intimate. We had become fast friends. I felt I could tell her anything. There were many similarities in our lives yet our lives were so different, too! I felt a connection I could not explain, and every time I read a message from her I felt invigorated to keep moving forward. We both held a passion for helping others out there with this diagnosis and we were both sure that "everything happens for a reason," as we had stated many times in just the few days since we had first started corresponding with each other. Then, on August 9th, I received a lengthy email from Mel. We were still in the stages of getting to know each other's lives. But the last sentence of this particular email was the turning point for me. Mel wrote:

"Oh by the way, my birthday is also in March. March 12th. When is yours?

Sincerely

Melanie"

I was speechless. And to get a better picture of my reaction, this was my response:

"Mel, no crap here, I just read your letter and my husband was sitting here with me. We both almost fell off our chairs. There are many, many similarities between us, but the most bizarre, and I am not kidding...My birthday is March 12th, 1968. Oh my GOD! I think this is so great!!!! It's late. I will write more tomorrow. Take care and I hope you are having a fabulous weekend.

Colleen"

The connection had been completed and the bond had been forged. We didn't know it yet, but the "Sisterhood Movement" had been born.

Chapter 2

The meaning of this diagnosis had changed for me dramatically. I was always taught to look for something good in everything. What was the lesson to learn? What was the purpose? As Mel and I continued to connect and communicate, it was just a few days when she wrote this:

"Hi Colleen,

I just wanted to say hi. I read your email while I was eating my dinner. I swear reading your emails are like you are reading my own thoughts. I will tell you more about that tonight when I email after work. There is something so powerful going on here. The funny thing is I made copies of all our emails last night and started a folder to keep them in. I don't know why, but I thought it was important to do that. I hope you're having a great day.

Till later tonight,

Mel

(I so look forward to your emails as well) "

I remember thinking how incredible this all was and my response to her was:

"Mel, I am waiting patiently. I think there is something going on here too. Let's figure it out.

Colleen"

The really funny thing is that I had started a folder for our communications as well. Great minds, right?

Many things were to transpire concerning the "Sisterhood Movement" over the next year, but my life was about to change again.

It was August 2008, and I had a clear PET scan in July. But by the end of the month, I was not feeling very well. Very tired again! I went to the gynecologist, as I was due for an exam. She said I had a bacterial infection and put me on a course of antibiotics. Of course! I had an infection. No wonder I felt like crap. In the back of my mind, I must admit, I felt there might be something more sinister going on. I pushed that thought way back and kept looking forward to all the emails from Mel. The doctor said it was just a bacterial infection, after all, nothing to worry about. A few days later Mel emailed me with the news. We had another "sister" or "comrade', as we first called them.

Back in the beginning of our communications, Mel had asked me if I had any ideas for a name if we started a website or something. A website? I could do that. A website for women with this cancer. A place for other women feeling alone and isolated. We could start with that. We had been discussing and researching the idea of a nonprofit. Mel had even bought a book called "Nonprofits For Dummies". It seemed like such a daunting undertaking, at the moment, with really only two of us. But a website was doable. On September 2nd of 2008, I emailed Mel with the news. We had a website up and running. It was called, "Cancer Comrades". The premise of the website was that any women suffering this diagnosis could come to our site. They would be matched, hopefully with someone close to their geographical area, so that they would have someone like Mel and I did. What ended up happening was that once we started communicating with these people, sisters and their supporters alike, we found we couldn't stop. We were supposed to let them go and maybe check in from time to time, but the ultimate goal was to help them find support and move on to the next person that needed us. In a short period of time, we had reached women from all over the world. Within a year we would lose some of them. We were juggling with the emails and phone calls. We had more than 16 "sister/comrades" and supporters and the daily toll was almost too much. We felt as if we were letting them down when a week would go by and we were unable to check in with one. A series of events eventually led to directing these women and their supporters to connect with us on Facebook. From Facebook, we were able to easily keep in daily contact with our comrades and we were also able to share more information freely, and even invite them into a closer look at our lives. We became friends.

During the fall I was still battling a supposed bacterial infection and the fatigue was worse than ever. In late November, I was sure I felt what I would describe as a small rock inside the opening of my vagina. Oh, I was done with the gynecologist. Obviously this was more than an infection. I called my radiation oncologist and found that, unbeknownst to me and to my dismay, he had left the practice just the day before. More worried about what was going on with me than why he was gone, I asked to have my PET scan scheduled. It now had been 4 months since my last one. Why hadn't anyone called from his office to schedule? It was an automatic thing. Every three months, like clockwork. I would later find out it was due to the reasons behind why my radiation oncologist was no longer with the practice. I loved him. He was my saving grace in all of this. I also had a great respect for my oncologist, but my radiation oncologist and I had hit it off on a level beyond patient/doctor, and I truly felt he had saved my life. This time it would be my oncologist who saved me...he was willing to fight against the odds. There were about three weeks between the time I first called the radiology office with my symptoms to the time I finally gave up and called the oncologist. Of course, now he was on vacation until after the first of January, and I would have to wait. No one seemed as concerned as I. I knew deep inside what was going on, but since the doctors didn't seem worried with what I was presenting, maybe I shouldn't be either. Couldn't that hard spot be radiation damage after all? In December, the "rock" grew bigger and there was no discounting it was there. It was Christmas, and although I should have pursued it, I didn't feel like it. Let me enjoy the holidays.

January was here and it was time for me to take this lump seriously. I called my oncologist and I was at a PET scan the next day. I got my results that afternoon, by myself, reading them while sitting in my truck. I never liked to wait for the results. The cancer was back. I was a little dumbfounded and dazed. I did not want to go through this again. Didn't they say there would be no cure if this came back? I would never be cancer free? Then why put myself through it? I had to. There was this nagging feeling in the back of my mind that kept me thinking, "this can't be it." I knew I was here for a purpose and I just couldn't fathom I had achieved it. No, I would not die. I would be cancer free again. I didn't "will" it to be so. It was something I just knew. I had surgery to remove my right ovary, as it had spread there. Then I started chemo again. Same as the last time, only my body really hadn't recovered from the last battle. This was hard. My hair fell out practically all at once, and I was so tired. But just as I had the last time, I went to all my appointments and handled everything the best I could, by myself at home. I finished chemo in July of 2009, and I could feel that at least the lump was gone. But the PET scan was showing a spot somewhere in the vaginal cavity. Unsure exactly where, as radiation had made things unrecognizable, I had an Abdominal Hysterectomy in September 2009. Today, almost four years later, I am still cancer free.

By this time, we were still getting members on Cancer Comrades and people were finding us on Facebook, through others members on Facebook, and through some articles I had written and posted on the web. It wasn't a good thing that we were growing, but it was a good thing these women and their supporters had a place to go. Without these members of our Sisterhood, I do not know what I would have done. They prayed for me, they wrote letters and sent me cards. They kept on top of my treatments and surgeries and I could hear the virtual battle cry to have hope and survive throughout the miles that divided us. I also became even closer to Mel at that time. I may be wrong, but I think me being sick again made her very upset. Possibly she worried hers might come back, but I truly feel she was concerned that I might not make it. I can't put into words what is between Mel and I, or at least not on my side of it. She is everything I wish I could be. She is the fish in the Pisces symbol, swimming the direction of the tide in calmness and prudence, while I am the fish in the symbol, swimming against the tide in excitement and emotion. She gets me and brings out the best in me. Without her I could have never found the peace and calmness to fight this a second time. But I did! I did it with the help of our "sisters", my loving family and supportive friends. I did it because of Mel! In the beginning of this journey for me, I prayed to God one night, asking him for 10 years. If he gave me 10 years, I would go peaceably with him after that. It's now been almost 7 years. I hope he is open to negotiation.

Melanie's story, in her own words:

My name is Melanie Cummings. At the age of 43 years, I was busy working and living my life. I woke up on the morning of May 1, 2007, just like every other morning. But this morning would be very different. I had no idea, in a few short hours, how my life would be changed forever.

Going back 6 months prior, October 2006, I had begun to have vaginal bleeding. I had not had a period in a very long time. I don't even remember when my last one had been. I just thought, "Yeah, I am menopausal." I was just happy not having them. I would make excuse after excuse as to why I was bleeding. Before I knew it, 6 months had passed since the bleeding began. I really am not sure what prompted me to finally make an appointment. As an adult, I had never liked going to the doctor, especially the gynecologist. I think I am probably like a lot of women who feel the gynecologist visit can be uncomfortable and embarrassing. I look back and all I can think is how incredibly stupid I had been. The choice I made to ignore my symptoms could have cost me my life.

The morning of May 1, 2007, I had a follow-up appointment with the gynecologist, Dr J. I was very nervous that morning. Looking back, I am not really sure I knew what to expect. Dr J had done an exam 2 weeks prior, and she had found a mass that she thought might be a polyp. She did a biopsy and asked me to come back in 1 week. She brought up cancer that day, but I tried to put that in the back of my mind. My original follow-up appointment had to be rescheduled because my results were not in yet. I really was not alarmed that the results were not in yet. I think I must have been in denial. My follow-up was rescheduled for May 1, 2007, at 11 am. Well, to say the least, I was very annoyed. I had plans to be out of town with some family that day. My aunt had been diagnosed with Melanoma and I wanted to have a fun few days with her. I made the decision to cancel my appointment and reschedule for a later date. I knew I should not have canceled my appointment but I wanted to go on my trip. The nerves set in and something was not feeling right. I had been Googling about vaginal bleeding. I worked in a hospital as an Ultrasound Tech and why it had never dawned on me what could be wrong seems crazy to me now. I am not sure why, but I called the doctor back and took my original appointment for May 1st.

So d-day was here. I had to be at my appointment at 11 am to get results of my biopsy. It seems funny to me that I can remember the time all these years later. I had been keeping a secret from everyone about all the vaginal bleeding and that I had a biopsy. I am a very private person and don't discuss these kinds of things with anyone. A few days prior to May 1st, my mom kept hounding me because she knew something was wrong with me. So, finally, I blurted the words out of my mouth that I may have cancer. My mom knows me, and when I don't talk it's only because I am sick or upset. I had been very quiet and she knew something was wrong. The morning of my appointment she had said, "Do you want me to go with you?" I said. "No, I will go by myself." I am glad I was alone for my appointment. It would give me time by myself to absorb all the information

I would hear that morning. Really, all I was worrying about was that Dr J had said she might have to take me to the operating room. That would prove to be the least of my problems.

I made my way to Dr J's office that morning. I sat quietly in an exam room, waiting for her to come in. Dr J was very somber when she came into the room. I can remember as if it were yesterday, hearing the words come out of her mouth, "I am sorry. You have CANCER." Then came the next hit, "It's called Neuroendocrine Cervical Cancer, and it's not good." I would soon learn it also goes by another name, Small Cell Cervical Cancer or SCCC. I was familiar with the words Small Cell. My Dad had died 3 years prior from Small Cell Lung Cancer. I can't help but feel my dad was with me that morning, as May 1, 2007 would have been his 68th birthday. Of all the days of the month, this would be my diagnosis day. I felt it was my dad letting me know he would watch out for me and see me through this journey I was about to begin.

I left the doctor's office that day with instructions to be at my primary doctor's office in 1 hour. Two days later, I had an appointment with a Gynecological Oncologist named Dr H. I went to my car and cried my eyes out. I begged God not to do this to my mother. My mom had been through so much. I did not want her to have to bury a child. I called my mother and broke the news to her then I called just one friend. After that I was just not up to talking to anyone. Thank God for my mother. She was in fighting mode and handled everything from appointments to referrals to making sure I ate. She would later tell me she never believed anything was going to happen to me. I felt the exact opposite way. I just wondered WHEN I was going to die.

Probably the biggest mistake I made in the early days after my diagnosis was going on the computer and searching for information. The phrase "POOR PROGNOSIS" still haunts me, to this day.

Those first few weeks were very tough. You cannot imagine how hearing the words, "you have cancer," could cause so much physical pain. But I ached so badly. One day I got down on my knees and begged God to help me. I did not even want to get out of bed. He heard my prayers and, about 3 weeks after diagnosis, I returned to work. I worked throughout my whole treatment. I look back now and I really cannot believe I worked through all my radiation and chemo. But I felt I would rather be productive than feel sorry for myself. My co-workers and boss were really great. I was not going at my normal speed, due to side effects of treatment, and they would just pick up the slack for me.

I was on a chemo/radiation combo. I would do radiation every day before work. Friday was Chemo Day, along with radiation. That would be the only day I would take off work. I would spend most of the weekend in bed and then I would get back up on Monday morning and do it all over again. I did it that way for over 6 weeks! Internal radiation began immediately after external radiation was completed. I was horrified after my simulation day, when I found out what this part of treatment would entail. I am so grateful, due to circumstances, that God had sent me an amazing doctor to get me through this part of my journey.

I knew from the first time I met Dr P, that he was meant to be my radiation doctor. He always has kept me informed and been honest. From Day 1, I always knew he wanted what was best for me. He went above and beyond to make me as comfortable as he could. It also helped when I learned he was the brother of one of the residents at the hospital where I worked. I knew I was in good hands. I felt sorry for Dr. P because I was one nervous wreck, out of my mind with fear, cancer patient. Thank you Dr. Patel. You have gotten me through some of my darkest days.

Treatments ended mid-July 2007, and after nothing but doctor visits and treatment for 3 months, I heard the words, "See you in three months!" I am not sure why, but I was freaked out. I counted down each day of treatment, wanting it to all be over, and now that it was all over, panic would set in big time. I was supposed to go on with life like nothing had ever happened. But there was one small problem. "Poor Prognosis" was hanging over my head. How do you not worry and not think about dying when you know all this information about this type of cancer? Every day I cried myself to sleep in fear. Would tomorrow be the day this journey would take a bad turn?

It was time for a well-earned vacation. Off to Florida I flew with my niece, Amanda, and sister, Toni, in August 2007. I had never earned a vacation more than this one. It was on this trip, sitting by the pool, that we came up with this crazy idea to try and go somewhere, on an airplane, every 4 weeks until Christmas. I thought, "What the heck? I am down for this!" I rationalized in my head, either I am going to die and have no money left or I will live and make more money.

The very next month we headed to Disneyworld. I would later learn my sister, Toni, knew how serious this cancer was and I think she wanted to make sure she spent as much time as she could with me. We were having such a great time traveling. We would be home a few weeks and head off again. I do believe the traveling saved me from losing my mind. After a few trips, we said, "What the heck? Let's try and see if we can do this for one whole year!"

In November, sitting in Florida again, we hatched our next plan which we called, "Canceling Christmas for Key west." No presents, just go and have family time and make memories. My sisters, Vicki and Toni, along with my brothers-in-law, Bob and Tony, and my niece, Amanda, headed to Key West with just a few weeks' notice. This would be the first of 5 Christmases in a row spent in Key West. Christmas 2011 was our 5th Christmas in Key West. We have made memories to last a lifetime and I feel so grateful we had the chance to do all those trips. We have learned how precious life is and made wonderful friends along the way. I think, after all was said and done, I traveled somewhere each month, for 15 months straight!

After treatment ended, the first year consisted of visits with my radiation oncologist and gynecological oncologist every 3 months, along with PAP smears, CAT scans and PET scans. I was just working, traveling and trying to forget about cancer, but it was always there. It was like the elephant in the room.

I recall a specific trip in Feb 2008. It was another trip to Florida. Yes, I love Florida!!!! I was sitting in the Ft. Lauderdale Airport waiting to fly home. It was packed with people everywhere. I had been sitting with some young women who were quite annoying and I had to move my seat. I ended up sitting next to a physician from Michigan. We talked for hours while waiting to fly home. I began to *tell her my story and why I was traveling. By now, I was used to the look I would get when I would meet people with a medical background and I told them I had SCCC. I called it the, "poor girl" look. It's like they knew I was going to die. I was always careful about the questions I asked doctors because I knew I had to be willing to live with the answers. This would end up being a very important night for me. I am not sure what came over me that night, sitting in the airport. I had never asked my own doctors if anyone had survived this cancer, I'd just assumed everyone died because of the poor prognosis I had read on the Internet. The nice doctor from Michigan had told me she had 1 patient in 25 years with SCCC. Before I knew what was happening the words were coming out of my mouth, "Is she still alive?" I could not believe what she said next, "Why, yes. It's been thirteen years."*

I could not believe it! There was someone who had survived! I have never doubted for one second that God had placed her there for me that night. He knew I needed to hear her message. I would take that information and hold it very close to my heart. One survivor meant hope for me. For the first time in 9 months I felt a glimmer of hope.

Although I was surrounded by my loving family and friends, I quietly felt all alone. I cried myself to sleep every night, worrying when this cancer was coming back and if I am I going to die. I felt so alone.

I had sworn off searching on the computer for stuff about SCCC. I am not sure why, but in August 2008, I starting searching again. Maybe it was because I prayed I would find something other than "Poor prognosis." I am not sure what I was searching for that night, but I had stumbled upon a cancer website called Cancer Compass. I had also seen this site the year prior. You could search by your type of cancer and find other people, with the same diagnosis, who communicated on the site. Most of the posts were a few years old. It was like the people would just disappear. I would later learn they had died. This particular night, I found a post from a mother whose daughter was newly diagnosed with SCCC. I decided I would send her a message and let her know I had been diagnosed 15 months prior and I was doing well.

I had no idea how life-changing the decision I made to post that night would be for me. A few nights passed after I had posted my message. I came home from work and was checking my emails. I had an email from a woman named Colleen Marlett. My first thought was, "Who the heck is Colleen Marlett? Why is she sending me an email?" I opened the email and, to my surprise, she was a woman who also had SCCC. I was overjoyed, to say the least. Colleen was diagnosed 9 months before I was. We were both thrilled to have found each other. It was like Christmas. In the beginning, we both were typing our hearts out. For the first time since my diagnosis, someone knew exactly how I was feeling. I could not wait to get home and read the next email from her. A few days in, I recalled Colleen saying her birthday was in March. I sent off an email to her to let her know my birthday was March 12th. To my surprise, I received an email back and learned that Colleen and I shared the same birthday! I almost fell off the chair when I read her email!

It did not take us long to realize there was a purpose that we found each other. Just a few short weeks after we came together we decided we did not want any other women *diagnosed with Small Cell Cervical Cancer to ever feel as alone as we had. So we came up with the idea to buddy women together, kind of like having a pen pal. It had meant so much to us and we wanted that for the other women living with SCCC, too. We wanted our website to be called Cancer Buddies, but the name was taken so we chose Cancer Comrades. Before I knew it Colleen had our website up and running. Our goal was to buddy women together. We would match them together and move on to the next match. I was so excited when the first woman found us. Her name was Shawna. I would learn about Shawna's family and friends. I can remember how excited she was that her sister in-law, Carol, was getting ready to have her first nephew, Evan. She was so excited when he was born. Shawna would live to see Evan's first birthday, but died a few months after.*

Many people would contact us over the next several months. We were supposed to match each person with someone and move on but, for some reason, we could not let go. Colleen and I both continued emailing each person that contacted us. At one time I was emailing 60 people!

We both realized something big was going to come from all of this. But, to be honest, we could have never imagined all that has happened the last 4 years. We had a dream that no women diagnosed would ever feel alone. I strongly believe that God has had His hand in every step of this journey. There are so many people that have joined The Sisterhood over the last 4 years. Each one bringing her talents, love, passion and hope to this special group of women. We, as a group, could not be where we are today if not for the efforts of so many wonderful people. We have our sisters and those who support us to thank for that. Colleen and I had a dream no women would ever feel alone again when diagnosed with SCCC. Maybe Colleen and I started the train with our dream, but many have joined along this journey. They have also had a dream and a passion to make a difference, as we had in the summer of 2008. The train ride was just the stepping off point to get us where we are today. All that has been accomplished would not have been possible without the efforts of so many people.

We began to have many women find us in those early days. About 6 months in, we would experience our first loss. I was devastated beyond words. I was curled up in a ball on my bed, bawling my eyes out. This would just be the beginning of many losses to come over time. Young women were dying and leaving behind many loved ones who were devastated by their deaths. Many times I have had to ask myself, "Why I am doing this?" Can I stand to watch one more young mother leave her babies behind? Or young women, just beginning life, never having a chance to become mothers. Gone way too soon. Somehow I dust myself off and continue on. I would be lying if I did not say it's very hard, at times. But I continue the fight for my sisters no longer here. I fight for my living sisters and I fight for the women who will be diagnosed in the future.

You begin to settle into a routine. Doctor visits and test time. I always get very nervous at test time. Some might call me cranky around these times, but the truth is I am always scared to death. You never stop worrying about this cancer coming back. Even after 5 years, I still worry all this time. I still get that sick feeling before a scan. Something I am not sure will ever go away.

About 6 months after connecting with Colleen, she got

devastating news that her cancer was back. I think it was natural to wonder, "Am I next?" Colleen worried about me, and how I would take the news. I was terrified for her and for myself. But I can recall Colleen telling me, just because her cancer came back does not mean that would be my fate. To be honest, I never thought she would survive.

I knew Colleen was in for the fight of her life and I would have to take a more active role in Cancer Comrades. Colleen needed to concentrate on getting through chemo. She would answer emails whenever she could and I would keep her updated on the sisters and let her know when we found someone new.

I could never shake the horrible fear I was going to die. I longed for my life BC (before cancer). Life was so easy then. I felt a great need to get things in order, so when the cancer came back, I would be ready. I wanted to make things easier on my family. I watched my mother having to go through all my father's stuff after his death, and I was determined I would make it as easy as I could for my family. So I got rid of everything I could.

I can remember asking Dr. P when can we worry a little less. He said, "When we get to three years we can worry less, and at five years I will be really happy." So I would count every milestone I could. Finally, I made it to the 3-year mark! For the first time I dared to think, "maybe I can survive this horrible cancer."

Since the beginning of my diagnosis, I've felt it is very important to share my story about my cancer journey every chance I get. Although my cancer was not the normal cervical cancer, I have a great opportunity to share my journey in hopes it will encourage other women to get their

PAP smears.

My life has changed forever because of my diagnosis. If I am to be truthful, the emotional and physical side effects have been very hard. I don't think any cancer patients would ever say they are grateful for their diagnosis, but I try to embrace and appreciate the many blessings and amazing people that have come my way because of my diagnosis. My Cancer Sisters and our supporters are some of the most amazing people I have ever met. They have only been brought into my life because of the diagnosis.

At some point Colleen said she had Myspace, so I decided to get an account as well. Not long after that, we heard about Facebook, and we both got an account there, too. We would soon learn some of our Cancer Sisters were also on Facebook. This was a great way to send a quick note and keep in touch with each other. We would do these long, private threads on Facebook, so all the sisters could talk together. We had some great conversations. We could share our fears and our victories. This would just be the beginning of what was to come.

Women continued to find us through our website, Cancer Comrades, and from articles that Colleen had written about her journey. In the early days the Sisters were Debbie, Shawna, Angela D., Kristi, Michelle, Colleen, Sharon, Kerri, Kimberly and some others. The early days also brought supporters like Sandy, Suzanne, James and a few others. We were a little group, and what we lacked in numbers we made up for in our hearts.

One of our sisters, Angela V., had joined our little group in January 2010. Toward the end of spring that year, Angela had an idea to start a private page for our sisters on

Facebook. Only those invited could be on this page and others would not be able to see anything written. Angela created the page and we all joined. We were all in one place now, so all the sisters would be able to get to know each other. It was our new home. I don't think anyone could have imagined how this idea to have a private page would become a game-changer in the fight against SCCC. Angela would bring many women she had found on Inspire and Cancer Compass to Facebook. This was just the beginning. Angela has done an amazing job helping women diagnosed with SCCC and LCCC to find their way to our group. She has kept things up and running and has never missed an opportunity to bring awareness to Small and Large Cell Cervical Cancer, since starting the page. My hat is off to you, Angela. I told her I would be her partner in crime anytime. Working together, we can make amazing things happen.

We were growing closer and closer as sisters as time was going by. Our numbers were increasing. Women can now find us at the beginning of their journey instead of feeling alone, as so many of us had felt. Along this journey we have lost many women to this horrible cancer. We cry and mourn our losses, but we come back to give our love and support and hope to those left behind.

I am amazed at the strength and faith our sisters show each and every day. We all have our moments and our sisters are there to pick us up and help us continue the fight. We all come from different places in the world, brought together because of a cancer diagnosis. Some might say this is just a cancer support group, but so many of us have formed amazing friendships, along the way, that will last a lifetime. I consider that one of the greatest blessings.

Our Sister Supporter, Jessica, is one determined women. I love the story she tells about wanting somewhere to donate money because of her sister, Jen's diagnosis of Small Cell Cervical Cancer. Because of Jessica's sheer determination, our fund at MD Anderson was formed. When no one was willing to research our rare cancer, we helped ourselves. I think we have surprised a lot of people along this journey. What we lack in numbers we make up for in our hearts and determination.

Our first project was having bracelets made to raise money for our fund. This was how the motto "Rare But There" was born.

In early 2011, the buzz began about a cancer conference for young people in New York in April. Angela asked if anyone wanted to meet in New York. I do believe that up until this point, none of us had ever met in person. I thought I would love the chance to meet our sisters. Over the next few months I went back and forth with whether I should go or not. I knew once I went, there was no going back. The people I had only known on the computer would now become real. My sister, Toni, encouraged me to go. She felt I would regret not going. Finally, with only a few weeks to go, I committed and bought my plane ticket. Toni flew to New York from Atlanta to meet the cancer sisters and attend the conference with me.

I am not sure why, but I was so nervous to meet the girls. I worried about what I would wear to what would we talk about. Angela had arranged for us to meet at a restaurant on Friday night for dinner. Our hotel was pretty close so we took off on foot to meet everyone.

I can remember walking though the door and immediately

seeing everyone at the table at the main entrance. There was no time to worry anymore. The greetings and hugs began. If I had to describe that night in one word, it would be "magical." The joy and love that filled that room was unbelievable. How could we have this love for people we had never meet before? But that is exactly what it was. The smiles were from ear to ear. For the first time ever, there were 9 women in the same room with Small and Large Cell Cervical Cancer. I don't think had that ever happened anywhere in the world before. I met 8 of my Cancer Sisters that night:

Angela V.

Jaclyn

Rosie

Becky A.

Debbie

Ally

Mona

Jen D.

We talked and laughed for several hours. I don't even remember eating that night, but I am sure we did. This night changed everything for us. We were very close to each other and there was no going back from this moment forward. We took pictures together that night. You would have thought we were famous with all the flashes going off! Besides the Cancer Sisters, many of us brought a supporter with us. The night was everything we could have hoped for and more. We attended the conference that weekend then headed back to our lives.

I think most of us who went to New York would later admit that we struggled after we got home. This was no longer just people we knew on the computer. We all had become very real to each other. I knew the odds were not good that all of us would make it, so we were opening our hearts up for pain. Many times I have had to ask myself if I could change things, would I still have gone to meet my sisters? And the answer is always the same. Without a doubt, YES!

We knew upon returning home we would plan do the conference again in 2012. The conference would be in Las Vegas 2012 and I purchased my plane ticket in August 2011. I was determined to be there, no matter what.

In August, I traveled to Minnesota to visit my sister's family. One of my Cancer Sisters, Rosie, lived very close to my sister, so we made plans to see each other. We went to the Minnesota Zoo to visit Rosie at work. Rosie took us on the train she drove and it was so nice to see her and hug her again. We also met for coffee before I returned home. Rosie had a cough at this visit that would not go away. She soon learned her cancer had spread to her lungs. My sister, Vicki, became friends with Rosie and her mom, Donna. I was grateful because Vicki would later be able to help Rosie when she needed it most. I know there was a purpose for meeting Rosie.

In November, I traveled to Chicago and had the chance to meet another sister, Candeese. The first thought I had when I saw her was how tall and beautiful she was. Her stepmom, Sabrina, joined us and we had a wonderful lunch and talked and talked. The fear I once had of meeting my sisters was now gone. Candeese was also coughing at lunch. My heart sank, as I knew what that probably meant. We made plans to meet again, as I would be back in Chicago for a doctor visit in December. We hugged and said our goodbyes. I was so happy we had lunch that day. It was a really great visit.

The end of November 2011 was the beginning of some very hard times for our Cancer Sisters. On Thanksgiving Evening 2011, we lost our sister, Ally. I had the great pleasure of meeting Ally in New York. She had sat at my end of the table, along with her sister, Katy, and boyfriend, Todd. We had such a great time talking. You could not have been in a room with Ally without knowing how special she was. Her life had just begun and now it was over. It was just heartbreaking. After Ally passed away her family and friends donated a lot of money to our research project, in memory of Ally. I was blown away how many lives she had touched. Ally, I think of you often and I know how proud you must be of your family and the Allyson Whitney Foundation, fighting for young people diagnosed with rare cancers. Sending much love to Barbara, Katy and Barri.

December 2011 was not any better. Candeese died and then Rosie followed, not long behind. I had met each one of these girls. Candeese and Rosie left their children behind. I had met Rosie's children back in August. None of this ever seems fair. No child should have to grow up without his or her mother. You feel so helpless with this cancer. But I also know, although it was a short time I had Rosie in my life, it was for a purpose. We got to meet her mom, Donna, in New York. I do believe my family is supposed to stay in Donna's life, along with Rosie's sweet babies. I look forward to many visits seeing Donna and the kids when I travel to see my sister in Minnesota.

I was struggling after the deaths of Rosie, Ally and Candeese. What am I doing opening myself up to all this pain? But, once again, I asked myself, would I change meeting them? And the answer always was, I would do it all again in a heartbeat. I feel very blessed that I had the opportunity to know these women, even if it was only for a short time. They were all wonderful and the greatest way I can honor their memories is to continue fighting to make a difference for women diagnosed with Small and Large Cell Cervical Cancer. It just makes me more determined than ever to help others and try and make a difference.

Since January is Cervical Cancer Awareness Month, we decided to bring in 2012 with a video to bring awareness to SCCC/LCCC. Every chance we get, we share our stories, in hopes that someone is listening.

We planned to head out to Las Vegas for the cancer conference at the end of March, 2012. Angela V. and I joined forces and we were determined to get as many sisters to Vegas as we could. I am not sure how we did it but we were able to help several sisters get there with financial and airline mile donations. We had 19 sisters, many supporters and our beloved Dr F., who is heading the research and fundraising project for SCCC/LCCC at MD Anderson, heading to Vegas. We bunked 3 and 4 in each room to make it happen. The money just came. We had a dinner planned on Thursday night, where we would meet some sisters for the first time. Seven of the 9 sisters who attended the New York conference were also coming to Vegas. Ally and Rosie had both planned on attending before they lost their battles. Angela and I worried about every detail. We wanted the *night to be perfect.*

On this trip I would finally get to meet Colleen, after almost 4 years of a friendship in the making. We had talked many times on the phone and sent many emails and messages on Facebook. Finally, we would be in the same room. She flew in Thursday afternoon and came rushing into the room because she was running late for our dinner. We hugged and hurried to get to dinner. I told her later, it almost felt like we had met before. It was not weird or awkward at all. Just normal, like we had known each other our whole lives. Friends forever!!

As it had happened in New York, the energy was so incredible in the room. Along with Dr F., we had sisters come in from Australia, Norway, Canada, and all over the United States. I think we had 40 people at dinner. Most of us stayed in the same hotel so we could have lots of time together. But it is never enough. We laughed and we cried together. I wish each sister could have the chance to meet at least one other. It was amazing meeting Dr F. He flew all the way from Texas just to meet with us and tell us about our research project. We feel very blessed Dr F. has joined our fight. He's just another gift in this journey. Our sister, Sandy, and her husband, Norm, had brought all of us new t-shirts and we had a few more gifts for our sisters. We had a limo bus ride after dinner and saw a few of the sights of Vegas. We had a great time. I shared a room in Vegas with Pearlie, Colleen and my sister, Toni. We stayed up every night talking and laughing. The first night we were up very late talking and snuck downstairs and ate burgers and pancakes at 3 in the morning.

I had to be up early to meet in Angela's room on Friday

morning. Kelly Rogers, our Cancer Sister Shawn Knutson's sister, and I had arranged some clothing donations for our sisters. All of our sisters would get a new outfit and jewelry. It was so fun watching the girls trying on clothes and just sitting around talking.

Friday night all my roommates went over to the Venetian Hotel to visit with Jamie and Brandon Cagle, another sister and her husband. We had a great time just being together, talking. Jamie and Brandon are 2 of the sweetest people I have ever met. Sadly, Jamie lost her battle just a few short months after Vegas. I feel very fortunate I had the chance to meet Jamie in person. She was one strong, amazing woman with a strong faith.

Saturday, we attended the conference in the morning and did a little gambling in the afternoon. Almost the whole group met for dinner again on Saturday night. This was the beginning of our goodbyes. We attended a comedy show that night. Later, Melinda and Mya joined us in our room and we sat up very late, talking. Melinda was one of our sisters who had traveled all the way from Australia, along with SCCC sister, Charmaine and Mya, a sister supporter. Mona is our sister who traveled again, for the 2nd time, from Norway with her husband to join our sisters.

On Sunday, some of us ate breakfast together, did a little gambling and had some pool time. Some more of the girls flew out on Sunday night, with the rest leaving on Monday night. Debbie and Becky came and spent the last of their time in Vegas with my family at our hotel.

The weekend went very fast and soon we were saying goodbye, one by one. The tears were flowing and we were all hugging. I feel very lucky I once again had an amazing *opportunity to meet my sisters. I cannot wait until our next meeting.*

My Cancer Sister, Debbie, and her daughter, Geneva, came to spend the night at my house in July. They drove 5 hours just for 1 night. They arrived and I had to break the news to them that we had no power. We made the best of our situation and headed to McDonald's for dinner. We sat up very late talking and laughing by flashlight. I feel so lucky to call Debbie my sister and friend. We were just happy to be together. We got to decorate undies for Panties on the Bridge together, we did a little shopping and had dinner before she had to head home. Very sad to say goodbye but I know it won't be long and we will see each other again. Debbie was one of our early sisters. She is one amazing, strong woman. She is always there with good advice and love and support. She is my sister and friend and I am so grateful she is in my life.

I had seen last year that a family in Ohio had started a foundation to bring awareness to gynecological cancers, after losing their beloved Jaymie. They hung underwear on the Purple People Bridge. I told my sisters if they made them I would hang them. I had 100 pairs of underwear and I headed out on my 5-hour drive to Kentucky. I was lucky because my Cancer Sister, Kristi, and her mom, Peggy, were meeting me there. I also met Stacy. She was Jaymie's sister. I was so glad I went. The afternoon was wonderful. Although it was horribly hot, we had a great time. We met many of Jaymie's family and promised we would be back the next year. Kristi, Peggy and I went to dinner after our afternoon. It was wonderful to have another chance to meet a sister and a supporter and enjoy being together. I look forward to getting to visit with Peggy and Kristi again next summer.

Becoming friends and sisters with women that have been diagnosed with SCCC/LCCC, from all over the world, has been a true gift and blessing. I know people outside our group don't understand our bond and that's ok. To be told you have a rare cancer and you have a poor prognosis is something most people will never be able to understand. All of us wish this had never happened to us, but we cannot change our diagnoses. We make the best of our situations and try to help each other on this journey. The sisters understand each and every thought and feeling we might have. We are there for each other in good times and bad. We celebrate the victories and we support each other when things our tough. We share our fears and there is always someone there to lift you up, night and day. We are there to help our new sisters when their journeys begin, or for a sister and her family when the end of the journey has come. We have a wealth of knowledge and experience and ready to share at the drop of a hat. We have a lot of love and compassion for each other and our families.

To all my sisters and our supporters: thank you for always being there for me and for showing me the beauty that comes with this journey.

Dr Michael Frumovitz, thank you for taking us under your wing. You are one amazing doctor and friend to our sisters. I know with you leading the charge we will make a difference in the future for women diagnosed with Small and Large Cell Cervical Cancers.

Pearlie, thank you for your friendship. You have taught me so much over these last few months. You have wisdom way beyond your young years. I am so grateful I had the chance to meet you in person. I will cherish Vegas and the time we spent together always in my heart. It breaks my heart that I now must prepare myself that your journey will soon be over. I am not sure how I do that, as I am sure you are feeling the same way. I know we will meet again one day and I will always hold hope in my heart for a miracle for you. As with Rosie, I know there is a purpose that you came into my life. I know I am supposed to stay connected to your mom, Nina, and your children. I pray each day for your peace and comfort and your healing.

Xoxo

To my friend and sister, Colleen, I never would have survived the last 4 years without you. You have been an amazing friend and sister. I am very proud of you for the person you are and this project you dreamed of. As we prepared to work on this book project, we talked many times about how we could never find the original post that led us to find each other. As I sat at work one night

I decided to search again. I signed on to my Cancer Compass account. I saw there were some messages. I saw one from 2008 and decided to click on it. I was blown away. There in front of me, after 4 years, was the message I posted that led us to find each other. As I sat and read the message, what shocked me even more, was the fact it was 4 years to the day and 1 hour shy from the exact moment I had originally posted the message. We have gone through so much over the last 4 years and here we are, still standing. Thank you for all the countless hours you have spent at the computer working on this project - and all the other projects - so we can raise a little money for our research project and bring awareness to help women diagnosed with SCCC and LCCC. Thank you for riding the ride with me.

xoxo

Mel

Chapter 3

At about this time on the journey of our sisterhood, we had 20 or so women on our private Facebook page. They were mostly sisters, but we had a few supporters as well. We were getting ready to ring in 2010. We had been making a go of it as a group, able to post in real-time through threads, and the sisterhood was strengthening every day. January and the New Year would bring our group a new sister who would use her vision and "know-how" to change our path. She would join us, with others, in this fight and take us on the natural progression that we needed to follow in order to fulfill what we had set out to do in the first place. Even more women were now finding us on Facebook, through other members of the group, and still through the Cancer Comrades website. But we really didn't have a home.

One of our sisters and long-time survivor, Kimberly, who had come to us from Cancer Comrades, had recently met a woman who had only been diagnosed in November 2009, and was still going through treatment. Her name was Angela. From all I could see, this woman was on a mission of her own to not only survive this disease, but thrive through it, spread her message and reach out to those in her same situation. She was already on Facebook so I messaged her:

"*January 10, 2010*

Colleen Marlett

   SCCC

Hi Angela. My name is Colleen Marlett and I am a SCCC survivor. Kimberly Telleria sent me a friend request for you and I would love to connect. Sending you best wishes, lots of prayer and strong energy."

Within minutes I received a reply back:

"January 10, 2010

Angela Van Treuren

HI Colleen! Great timing! I was just getting ready to close down my Facebook when I saw I had a message. I start my 3rd round of chemo a week from Monday. They are saying we only have to do 4, so I'm almost done!!! YAY!! As you know it's certainly been a roller coaster. I would love to hear your story. When were you diagnosed? What was your treatment?

I saw there is a group on here for SCCC supporters and survivors but it's not a very active group. I may start a group just for us girls who have been through it/are going through it. Being that it is so rare, it's so awesome (as weird as it sounds) to find others who "understand".

I am keeping an online journal as well...www.caringbridge.org/visit/angelavant

Thank you SO much for reaching out!

Much Love, Angela"

I was elated when I got the message and, of course, I went

right to her blog so I could read all about her story. I could tell she was a kind and gentle soul who longed to share her experiences. She put herself out there so others with this diagnosis could find her and never feel alone. Her mission and passion clicked with what Mel and I had set out to do. But Angela was hungry and her tenacity brought women to us from other cancer sites, such as Inspire, and we were growing and growing. There was a crossover. Some women she would find and, at about the same time, some of the same women were finding us on Facebook through the website. Angela was full of great ideas and was always sparking conversations between us all as to what our next step might be. I remember reading one of her early postings to me. I got a true sense of her faith and connection to God. I knew she had been sent for a reason and that if God truly did work miracles, he was probably working through her for us. The email read:

"Thank you again so much for sharing your story! It means so much!

I am glad that we started with the chemo first, especially given that they already removed the tumor. I have so much hope and like you, know in my heart I will be here to live…there is just that level of fear and frustration knowing it could pop in again for a visit.

I give God 100% of the glory for the miracles that have already happened in my journey and my life. My faith and love for Jesus has grown clearer and more focused in this and for that I will forever be grateful!!

I am soooo not looking forward to next week. Chemo weeks are the worst but just 2 more rounds to go!! yay!!!

Be strong, you are in my prayers!!

Much Love, Angela"

The second paragraph;"I give God 100% of the glory..." is what solidified it for me. I knew she wasn't in this for self gratification, but for a bigger purpose. This movement was beyond any one person. I know Mel felt it too, but we were still only scraping the surface of what Angela would do for The Sisterhood.

From January 2010 to June of 2010, the sisters continued to have conversations through threads and posting with each other. Angela started a thread on May 28th, 2010 that included 17 women altogether. It read:

"May 28, 2010

Angela Van Treuren

    new SCCC sister....

Hi ladies, I hope this email finds you all doing well, feeling good and being blessed! We have a new SCCC sister and comrade that I will be sending out friend suggestions to you for. Her name is Jessica Barnett Lance. She was just diagnosed in April and has just completed her first round of chemo. I told her about all of you and she is excited to "meet" you. I just wanted to give you the heads up so you can welcome her with open arms when you see the friend suggestion.

There are 2 others that I am waiting to hear back from as to whether or not they are comfortable being introduced to the masses. haha. One is a survivor of almost 10 years. I believe and another is a current fighter. I will keep you posted on those two.

Love you all.....Angela"

As she found these women she would introduce them to all of us, as we did when they came to us from the web site or emails. For this being such a rare cancer, we were finding more and more sisters. If they were out there and alone, Angela would find them. The thread continued for several days as we talked about the fact that we were growing. What would do next? How could we get medical research involved? Discussions like that were flowing as we commented on losing 4 of our sisters in the prior four months. Here are a few of the comments posted to give you an idea:

"June 2, 2010

Melanie Cummings

   I think DR Finkler could use all of us as research. I am game for it !!"

"June 2, 2010

Colleen Marlett

   Me too"

"June 2, 2010

Kerri Alvarez

   Let's do this sistas.....need any help let me know..."

"June 3, 2010

Debbie Coulson Whyet

   Wondering if we should try to arrange a meeting or conference call to brainstorm or come up with a plan of action!!

I'm willing to travel"

"June 4, 2010

Colleen Marlett

   Well ladies, I think Debbie might be onto something. It's a good place to start. All of us together should be able to come up with something.

When Mel and I started Cancer Comrades two years ago, we did it so other women could find each other and never feel alone and isolated like we did. But, once we exchanged emails and heard someone's story, we couldn't let go of them. Here we are, two years later, with this wonderful group of women, being forced to let go of some of our comrades anyway. I watched the video slide of Kristi and I am not willing to watch or read anything like that about any of us again. She wore a pair of snowflake earrings in the pictures. I have the same pair. We are connected in more ways than we will ever know. If we can't make a difference for ourselves, then who can?

I don't know what the first step is. I do know that nothing is being done to save us from this horrible disease. We don't truly have cervical cancer, as nothing about this disease works the same except for the fact that the origination point happens to be the cervix. I had someone say to me, "Oh, I had cervical cancer. They just froze off the bad cells." Yeah, not working for me. I've also had countless people ask, "Why didn't they just give you a hysterectomy and be done with it?" Really? No one has any idea of the destruction of Small Cell originating in the cervix. They have no clue how staggering the numbers for fatality are and I am tired of sitting back and watching this disease pick one off and then skip over to the next. I know that is the way cancer works in general, but this is a 50/50 shot with us and something has to change, even if it's just to get a set protocol for treatment.

Let me know what you all think and then let's figure out how to do a conference call with all of us."

"June 4, 2010

Jaclyn Wright Guthmiller

Hi all,

Great discussions!

If we wanted to have a conference call, we could possibly use Skype to conference in people (which should be free if you are on your computer & have the program downloaded) otherwise, I am sure there are inexpensive conference call options available.

I have an article that my oncologists used as a starting point for my treatment. I will scan it in and send it on if anyone is interested. It is based on clinical trials from a few years ago (so it is a bit dated). I personally don't like reading all of the facts/figures in great detail because each person is different. I don't focus on the percentages because they are not real encouraging. But at the same time, we need to start somewhere to get those percentages of survival up!

Colleen, you are so right that small cell is very different than the squamous cell or adenocarcinoma types of cervical cancer. In my case, the tumor was a mix of all 3 types (neuroendocrine, adenocarcinoma and squamous cell) and mine was determined to be non-small cell (after a 2nd opinion). My onc discussed with us how each of the 3 types of cells would react differently with the various chemos. Because the majority of the tumor was neuroendocrine, in the end, I was still treated as if I had small cell using the article as a template for treatment, as there is no protocol for treatment for what I had. But at least my onc knew what type of cells he & I were dealing with.

I agree that it would be great to have a set protocol for treatment, as it sounds like each of us probably had a different treatment schedule, types of chemo, surgery first or last, etc.

I'm in for whatever the group decides to do - calls, emails, meet, etc."

"June 4, 2010

Kerri Alvarez

I hear you ladies. On more than one occasion I've heard people say, "ohhh I have had that." But they don't know that what this group of ladies has/had is a deadly cancer that acts faster than the type you can freeze off (not that that is not scary in itself), but this small cell is a very dangerous fight for us who go through it. Small cell of the cervix is rare and aggressive and we women have to go through much more than most people think. The internal radiation and external, the chemotherapy and the surgery and suffering that come along with it. There is so much in this fight. I pray that others can understand that this is not just an easy breezy process. I believe that we take on a lot in this fight. I hope that we all can show the world how much this is affecting women and that this is growing and growing. The numbers are getting higher. We need more research, more help to find out more about this. I love all of you sisters and hope to make a difference somehow, some way. You all are in my prayers and if I can be a help to anyone, please let me know. Love and respect, Kerri

Kerri Alvarez"

"June 4, 2010

Michelle Planten

My gyn oncologist started a foundation for gynecologic research. It's called Up The Volume Foundation. Check out the website at www.upthevolume.org. It would be great if we could get the great doctors together like Dr. Finkler in Orlando, and my Dr. Silver, and any others, maybe at MD Anderson or something. Anyway, I'm up for a conference call, if that's what we decide to do."

"*June 4, 2010*

Melanie Cummings

WE need to do something."

Our Angela, with ideas and the tenacity to see them through, came up with and delivered the next step in the natural progression of this journey. She posted:

"*June 4, 2010*

Angela Van Treuren

Wow......I love you all!!! I think we should totally try to get together, at least on a conference call to start, and put together some thoughts, brainstorm a bit and then maybe when we have some "action" items. We can meet wherever those action items may need to take place (like an MD Anderson or SKM)? What do you think? Like Jaclyn said, Skype works great! There are also some freebie conference call lines...I will do some checking out and let you know what I find out.

PS....We have another lady. I am going to send suggestions for. Her name is Mona. She was diagnosed 5 years ago. Had a recurrence 3 years ago and has been healthy for 2 years. She is in Norway.

Is there a way to add people to the recipient list of a thread or do we need to start a new one? Should I start a new group that is private to allow us to discuss without having to start new threads when we add a new comrade? I can start it and make you all admins. Let me know what you think....."

True to her nature, which is lucky for us, this was her next action:

"June 4, 2010

Angela Van Treuren

 So...I was on a mission tonight and went ahead and started a new group page. I will send you all invites....

You will see on the discussion tab of the group there is a thread to remember those we have lost. There is also a thread for us each to post our stories. It is a private group so only people we invite or "approve" will be members, so we can be honest, but the stories will help us as we try to get the attention of doctors and researchers, etc. I also found a couple free conference call sites that I will update you on. But...we can use this group page to really keep our discussions moving forward.

PS...I have my first 3 month follow up appointment on Monday. I will chat with my oncologist to see what she thinks about any directions we could maybe go in.

Love, Angela"

Small Cell Carcinoma Cervix Sisters United, known today as Small/Large Cell Carcinoma of the Cervix: Sisters United, was created!!! Our Facebook group was alive and well. We were all so excited and so happy to have a home! Quickly, all the girls joined. Angela brought in the women she was finding. Mel and I brought in the women finding us on Cancer Comrades, and really, all the ladies joined in and the mission that "no women would ever be alone in this fight" had just taken off like a rocket. How lucky were we that Angela had come to us 6 months ago? In the time since then, you can only imagine the things that have been accomplished by Angela and our group. We are so grateful that Angela used her passion and "know-how" to take us to the next level...and beyond.

Angela Van Treuren's story, in her own words:

"Angela E. Van Treuren

The Back Story

In every family there is always one kid who just seems to be the one to cause the most worry, who is always at the doctor and who, no matter what, will always be that troublemaker. Looking back I can say, without a doubt, that kid was me. Even though my long-term memory is so lacking, I can remember my time with crutches, casts, x-ray machines and visits to the urgent care or ER. When I was 17 and my mom thought I had a bad flu, of course it had to be appendicitis, leading to emergency surgery and weeks of recovery. I know that no one wants to have these ailments, but thinking about it now, what kid doesn't want a little bit of extra attention, right?

I grew out of my "clumsy" stage, I guess, and was able to start my adult life, doctor-free. As an 18 year-old who was just ready to take on the world, I left college after only a semester to start my career in marketing. I was eager and excited and I was blessed with a great opportunity, so off I went! I traded my flip-flops for high heels, and my jeans for professional slacks. I just knew I was on the fast track to success and, at the time, that is all I could have ever wanted. In my hometown of Fayetteville, North Carolina, there wasn't a whole lot of professional opportunity for growth. After a few years of getting my feet wet in Corporate America, I made the big move to New Jersey to keep my career going. Over the almost 4 years up North, I learned a lot about myself and I grew up in ways that, I didn't know at the time, were preparing me for what would soon be coming my way.

Probably my favorite thing in life has always been being a twin. People ask my sister and I all the time how it feels to be twins, and our response is always the same: it's our normal. We don't know what it feels like not to be. She is my best friend and after she moved to Washington State in 2000, after she got married, part of me was always missing and spread out across the 3,000 miles of distance between us. In 2005, I made the crazy decision to come out for a 2-week visit and just never left. I called my dad and he sold my furniture back East on Craigslist, put my boxes of stuff in his garage and I camped out on my sister's sleeper sofa for 6 months while I started to put together what would be my new life in Seattle. Here, I thought, is where my life would start to come together. I was 25 at the time. I was ready. And while I had no idea what to expect, I just had this feeling deep down that this place is where I would finally find the life I had always wanted.

It is pretty amazing to me that if we quiet our minds and our hearts, God is in there speaking to us so clearly. He is preparing us and when we trust in what He is saying, He will show us the way to hope. And that is where my story goes from here. It goes to a place full of so much hope, love and a journey that has been truly so blessed.

The Elephant In The Room

I was always very good about going to my annual check-ups with my primary care doctor. Preventative medicine is what it's all about, after all, right? Well, in 2009, I was a few months late from being one year on the button, but I wasn't concerned. I, after all, was living a successful life in a new Director of Marketing role, so who cared if my cholesterol would show up a little high because I was a few months late? That was my biggest health worry at the time. At 29, there couldn't be much else wrong. September 11, 2009, I walked into my primary care doctor's office. We laughed a little bit, had the normal annual pleasantries and she checked me out thoroughly. I recall being a little annoyed that day because they were running behind, which was going to make me late for a meeting.

One week, to the day, later I was driving in a major downpour of Seattle rain when my cell phone rang. I immediately recognized the phone number as my doctor's office. My heart sped up a little because I had seen in movies that they only call when something is wrong. So I put a smile on my face and answered the phone with as much joy as I could. My doctor's voice, somewhat shaky and quiet, was on the other end. She mentioned my cholesterol, which, yes, was a little high. But I knew she was beating around the bush. She then went on to say that something pretty abnormal had shown up in my PAP test and that she had already made a referral for me to see a specialist in Downtown Seattle. What followed was almost 6 weeks of tests, biopsies and a lot of guessing as to what was going on. On November 4, 2009, however, there was no more guessing. We got an answer, and it was an answer that none of us could have ever imagined.

I received a call from the specialist. Part of the conversation is a blur, but one statement that will live in my head forever is, "Angela, it's real cancer." Things seemed to go into hyper-speed after that. Within 2 days of the call I was scheduled for a PET scan, and just a few days after that I was to go see my oncologist for the first time. That was a doctor I had never thought I would have to say was treating me. An oncologist. Up until this point I had always known cancer doctors to treat either very young children or much older adults. However, at 29, I found myself with cancer, with a cancer doctor and quickly becoming entrenched into what I like to call "cancerland".

At the first meeting with the oncologist, her eyes were very serious and there was a layer of concern that hovered over her face. She indicated that the type of cancer I had was extremely rare: Neuroendocrine Small Cell Carcinoma of the Uterine Cervix. She had never personally treated it and barely anyone in her office knew about it. I immediately felt this familiar wave of panic. Here I was again, the kid causing the trouble; the girl with the rare cancer that nobody knew about. I found myself wishing I was 17 again and it actually was just the flu.

The initial tests showed what they called "disease" spread throughout my body. My sister and my father joined me at my second appointment with the oncologist and we conferenced my mom in on speaker-phone, as she still lived back in North Carolina. I will never forget when the oncologist looked at us and said we should probably talk about "the elephant in the room." I thought she was going to tell us how bad chemo was going to make me feel, or about how fast I would lose my hair. Instead she said that, statistically based on where the disease had spread, I probably had 6-12 months to live. I sat there realizing that she was telling me I may never see my 30th birthday. I may never get married or experience the joy of having children. I may never grow old to tell my grandchildren of this crazy day I was told I had cancer. All of a sudden those meetings I was late for back in September and that ladder climbing up Corporate America didn't seem so important. My sister asked me if I was scared and my response at the time was, "I'm annoyed." I was covering my fear and my tears with being positively annoyed that this was happening. I truly felt as though I was standing on the outside of my life looking in. To be sure this wasn't real.

A lot happened over the next 3 weeks. I had 4 surgeries to biopsy the "disease" throughout my body, my mom came to visit (which was amazing because she hates to fly) and most importantly I gave my life and my fight over to God. I knew He was truly The One in control of the life that I had always tried to drive. I knew that in this, He was going to have a purpose for me and I simply had to trust that His greater *purpose would be fulfilled. By His grace and mercy those biopsies ruled that the "disease" throughout my body was, in fact, not the cancer that they thought it was (it is sarcoidosis). My prognosis became much more positive and they re-staged me from a stage IV to a stage I.*

I went through the next 4 months in and out of chemo to treat the original tumor. I didn't have an appetite at all through treatment, except every few weeks on a Sunday morning I would crave pancakes. Something about that homemade taste and smell of melted butter brought me comfort. I still love the days I crave pancakes, a simple reminder of loving this life.

My follow-up scans have all been clear and I am almost 3 years from that original call to tell me that it was "real cancer." This journey and my world would not be the same without the fulfillment of what I believe to be the purpose, the bigger reason I was brought into cancerland. That reason is absolutely the Small/Large Cell Sisterhood. For anyone who ever feels alone in her illness, our story is one that brings about the reminder and realization that we are all in this together. We are never alone and even in the darkest moments, there is always hope!

Together, We are Now a Movement

When hearing the news that you have a rare cancer and no one else at your hospital has the same thing, it is a very alienating feeling. You do feel all alone. Then one day the loneliness changed to a glimmer of camaraderie. My aunt had found a discussion forum online on Inspire.com, the only one we could find that discussed our rare and aggressive form of cervical cancer. So I, being the social butterfly I am in any situation, logged on right away. No nerves at what I would find, no idea as to what would be awaiting me, just excitement at the possibility of talking with others who truly understood what I was going through.

I loved that early discussion thread, but I always felt the need to connect on a deeper level than that thread allowed. There was so much more I wanted to know about these women, who I was now considering my friends. In an age where social media is the lifeline to so much communication, there had to be a way for us to connect in a private group setting where we could really just bond, connect and reach others.

I had told some folks at my treatment center about a girl I had met online, Katie, whose sister, Jaclyn, from South Dakota, had come out the other side clean and clear and I was clinging to her story, believing that too could be me! The medical field knows how rare this cancer is and I know the thought that a few women could try to reach hundreds, from around the world, with this rare cancer was met with much skepticism. But we were determined! This cancer just doesn't know the strength of the women it had decided to mess with. We knew there were others out there and I asked God to show us how to reach those women so they would know they, too, were not alone.

So with the Facebook group, the Inspire girls and even some new sisters who had just found us, the Small Cell Carcinoma of the Cervix: Sisters United page was born. From there, momentum quickly picked up and we had the best thing any of us could have ever wanted...each other. We added Large Cell Carcinoma to our sisterhood, not long after the original start, in realizing the two are so closely related and have the same treatment paths and prognosis rates. The Small/Large Cell Sisterhood was born.

I remember the first sister we lost since first joining those discussions. Ally McLeod from London was a beautiful girl, only 27. She and I had shared many email conversations. Even in the end she said to me to keep fighting, keep going and never give up. Her smile and her words will live on in my heart forever, as we continue this journey.

In the spring of 2011, we made history happen when, for the first time ever, a group of Small Cell sisters met in person at Stupid Cancer's OMG Summit in New York City. We had 9 sisters from around the US, Norway and Canada. Our doctors were astounded and we were ecstatic. I will never forget the day we had to leave NYC. Those hugs will live on in my heart forever. We didn't know if we would ever see each other again, we didn't know how much longer some of us would live on this Earth, but we did know one thing: that we were a family.

That trip began a trend of sisters visiting each other in their travels and going out of their way when they would be nearby, just to get a hug. Sisters who live even remotely near each other began going to treatments with the other girls and bonding with their families.

One year after the first meeting we did it again. We met for the OMG summit, this time in Las Vegas. 19 of us showed up for this one and boy did we fill a room! Sisters from Australia joined in the fun this time, showing that our reach and our love know no boundaries or plane tickets. Sisters pitched in to help each other buy plane tickets, have spending money and share hotel rooms.

To me, this sisterhood is about reaching out in faith and hope and love. It is about fighting for those we have lost and those who are yet to come. One of our sisters once said, "Together, We are Now a Movement." I couldn't agree more. Alone we could never accomplish what this small, but mighty, group of women has done to raise awareness, money and support. But together we know that anything is possible.

Early on in my journey I ran across this quote that I believe is what all of us in the sisterhood have found:

"In the midst of winter, I finally learned that there was in me an invincible summer." ~Albert Camus.

As we walk this journey, the winter seems so cold, so dark and so lonely, but within each of us is a summer that burns so bright, so intently and so full of purpose. I have no doubt that the Lord's plan was to bring me to this group of amazing women. As hard as the journey sometimes gets, I will cling to that summer that He has given me inside to keep going to love my sisters and to never give up."

Angela continues to be a beacon of light, finding women from all parts of the world and connects us all together. Angela is an inspiration and an angel who has already earned her wings. Thank you, Angela, for who you are and all you do.

Chapter 4

One of the most amazing things about this journey and this group is the connection of women from all walks of life and from all over the world. Some of us were told that we would never meet another living soul with this diagnosis, but they were wrong. We have been fortunate enough to meet (both virtually and in person) women from Norway, England, Ireland, Russia, Germany Malaysia, Australia and Canada, to name a few. Here are a few stories, one from a woman in Norway, one in Canada, two in England and three from Australia. Mona (Norway), has already been mentioned in this story and is a long-time survivor and loving sister to this movement.

Mona's story:

I did not understand just how bad my diagnosis was until I went on the Internet to find out more about this cancer (my Dr. did not get into how weird and aggressive this type of cancer is). I cried every day for I do not even know how long. "Every time I looked at my kids, I just started crying." This is what Michelle, one of our passed sisters once wrote on the SCCC page.

It is not possible to describe with words what it is like to be told that you have a fatal cancer diagnosis. How it is to live with such a diagnosis. I know the feeling Michelle was describing. I remember the feeling when I was first told about my prognosis, how I first felt all the blood disappearing from my head. I got cold and completely overwhelmed; powerlessness came over me. But then after a while, I stomped the floor and became stubborn. Of course it took a while to get used to the thought of dying. There were days I just wanted to cry, and like Michelle said, every time I looked at my kids I was reminded of what would happen. My kids were going to experience things without me in the future! I would not be there at their graduation or their weddings. I wasn't going to be there to comfort them when they broke up with their first boyfriend or girlfriend. I wasn't going to be a grandmother. In short, they were going to live their lives without me!

I was first diagnosed in January 2005. I believed what I had was an innocent cell change and looked forward to a couple of days off from being a busy, working mum, when I went to the hospital to take some more tests. Being the optimist I am, it was not possible, even in my wildest fantasy, that it might be something serious with me. Even when I was told that it was malignant cancer, when I was operated on and put on chemotherapy, it did not occur to me how serious my cancer diagnosis was.

Just three weeks after I had finished the last chemotherapy, I was back at work again. I started to work part-time and within a year I was back at full speed, just like I had never been sick. I had only been back on full-time about six months when I got a call from my doctor. They had taken a sample of a lump I felt in my stomach, and it was now confirmed as malignant. I was told to come for a consultation, and to bring my husband. Then we knew something was really wrong!

I had to start chemotherapy right away. The cancer had spread, and they believed it was now in my lymph nodes. It wasn't possible to operate and chemotherapy was the only thing they could give me to hopefully slow progress, somewhat. But otherwise, there was nothing they could do. Bam! That was when I got that feeling that I described earlier. The blood disappeared from my head, I got ice cold and the complete emptiness, helplessness came over me. I cried for an hour then I was done with crying! Not that I have not cried since, of course I have, but that complete paralysis lasted no longer.

They say that you go through several phases when one experiences such shocks: anger, grief and acceptance. I went quickly into the acceptance phase. OK, when there is nothing you can do, you have to make the best of what you have. Who can I call? Who can fix this? Who can help me? No one can fix this. This is something you will have to deal with yourself!

At the beginning my husband and I were shocked. We tried to ask questions and dig for answers, but no one could help us. There was not much hope to find, and the message was clear: There is no hope!

After several months of chemotherapy, someone at the hospital found out that the tumor was not in my lymph nodes after all. It was in one of my ovaries, and suddenly it was possible to remove the tumor by surgery. After surgery, I got more chemo and then a whole year without anything, recovering again. The message was still clear: once it had spread, I was going to lose the battle in the end. The cancer cells had spread in my body and there was no treatment in this world that would be able to get rid of them.

To emphasize this, I got another recurrence a year later.

This time in the form of a water cyst filled with small cell cancer cells. It was removed by surgery. But this time I did not get chemotherapy. Because my body responds very poorly to chemotherapy, the doctors began to run out of options, and they chose this time to "keep the powder dry" until the next time. Then it may appear somewhere the tumors cannot be removed and, if so, the only alternative is chemotherapy to slow progression of the disease.

Now it has been seven years since I first became ill. During the past years, I have learned more about what kind of cancer I really have had: Small Cell Neuroendocrine Cervical Cancer. I have Googled and I have searched. But there is very little to find. And what I have found is usually not very encouraging. Some years ago, when I was fighting for my life, I found a research report from Korea. They had a case where a woman had lived for more than five years! I was so happy, and thought that if she can I can! It turned out that she had received similar treatment as me, so now my optimism was really justified! Later on I have learned that there are several other positive cases around the world.

Through my search I found someone else living with this cancer. One day, on a message board on Cancer Compass, I found other women writing and sharing their experiences. Finally I got the courage and wrote a message asking for help. This is what I wrote, after being told that I was going to die in 2007:

I am a 35 year-old woman from Norway. I was first diagnosed with neuroendocrine small cell cancer in january 05. At that time I had a small tumor on my cervix, this was removed by operation along with my uterus and surrounding lymph nodes. To be sure that I was going to get well I also went through several chemo treatments. Because of allergy, as well as low blood values I had to change treatment several times and ended up with carboplatin and Gemecitabin. After this the doctors said that my chances of getting cancer again was just as big as for anyone else....

Last November I discovered a large tumor in my stomach, this turned out to be a 10 cm large tumor spread to my lymphs. After this I have had a scan and it turns out to be "only" this tumor. Now I am back on the same chemo as last time, the doctors will not remove the tumor because they mean it is "already in my system" and they give me chemo to shrink it and hopefully stagnate it for some time. They are not able to give me any prognosis of how long I have got to live.

I have two small children (4 and 6) and this is a rather hopeless situation. I will do anything to see my children grow up!

Is there anyone who has had any experience with this kind of development? I have tried to search for help in other countries to see how they are treating this, but it is almost impossible for me as a private person to get hold of the people who know anything. Is there anyone that has been able to fight this back for a shorter or longer period, and if there is -how were you treated?

The answers I got to this and later messages made the start of lifelong friendships with some beautiful women all over the world. These women were the same ones that later on were starting the SCCC – Facebook page. A group of woman, growing larger every month, giving each other great support and help. Unfortunately, we have lost most of the women from the Cancer Compass message board, but some of us are still going strong and live our lives to fight this cancer.

Many people have asked me how I manage to stay so positive and live as normal as I do. My journey has been followed by many people, family and friends, and I eventually felt that I had something to tell. I started to write a diary on the web. I'm going to share a period of my life, my thoughts, my ups and downs, with you, in order to tell you my story.

Friday 10 October 2008

Today I decided to create my own website. After quitting working, I have plenty of time during the day, when the kids are at school. At the same time I feel that I have some thoughts and opinions that I want to write down, so I have made my own website!

Today the kids and I will go swimming. Maybe my husband will join us too, after work. I feel good. I've been home all day searching the Internet and looking after the cat, he has had surgery and has been sick the last days.

Yesterday I finally got a response from a doctor at the Swedish hospital in Gothenburg. I'm going to get an appointment and come to him for a "second opinion", still a little unsure when it will be, but I hope it will be soon...

I had no idea where this would lead, but I wanted to inform, there are many people out there who care about me and I felt this was a great idea to keep everyone updated on my situation. At the same time it had occured to me how difficult it is for many people to reach out in such situations.

I wanted to get ahead of them. The goal was that they should be informed of how I was doing, and not be afraid to contact us....

Monday 13 October 2008

The weekend was over in a fling... I had a great time at the swimming pool on Friday. I know that I need exercising! A friend of mine joined us, and she was kind to watch the kids while I was swimming. Saturday was like a marathon, with a very tight schedule. At first I was at a flea market, where I finally found a small desk that I'm going to paint and put in my daughter's room. Afterwards, the kids and I visited my parents. It has been a long time since last time we saw them! In the evening we visited some very good friends, it's always nice to spend time with them. On Sunday I slept late, I rarely do that anymore! Actually it was quite nice, and I know that I need to sleep more than before. Days with little sleep are much heavier than others. I don't like the feeling of being tired. It reminds me that the body no longer works 100%. When I then get to sit down I get too sensitive about every tiny ache, and then I get worried that something is wrong again...

Now it is nice the weekend is over so I can get a little time on my own. I am waiting to hear back from the Swedish doctor.

There is no secret that I, at times have been, and am very upset about my doctors' apparent lack of commitment. I have spent a lot of time to figure out how doctors in other countries work. In this process I have been in contact with two physicians who were engaged, internationally, in neuroendocrine cancer types. One of these doctors lives in Canada. He answered me nicely on my request, but unfortunately he could not contribute anything more than my doctors. The doctor in Sweden, who answered me, did not work primarily with the cervical variant, but a good colleague of his did. And they collaborated frequently in the treatment of this disease, so his colleague would certainly help me. This is the doctor I finally made contact with and tried to get an appointment with.

Wednesday 15 October 2008

Still have not heard anything from the Swedish doctor.... Last night my son and I were alone, my daughter was practicing gymnastics and my husband was swimming. We enjoyed ourselves with a movie and had a quiet and calm moment for ourselves. When I was getting him ready for bed, I put his pajamas in the dryer, so they would be nice and warm. When he put them on, he gave me a hug and said, "you think about everything, Mom." I believe he liked it....

I was with the physiotherapist yesterday. Going there today, as well. It's annoying that I have this lymphedema in my leg. After the first surgery, there were several lymph nodes in the abdomen that were removed and I have struggled with lymphedema. It makes my leg swell and become a little stiff. I have to wear compression sleeves all the time and to get lymphatic drainage at irregular intervals. But if that is the price of being well otherwise, I'll always be able to live with it...

Monday 20 October 2008

My son is not feeling well. He complains of stomachache and that he is tired. I know that he doesn't want to go to school, and think maybe that's why he is "ill". So today I *drove him to school. It resulted only in that the principal called after an hour and asked if I could come and take him home... I guess I felt a little guilty then...*

I feel pretty good, but I get scared about a pain I feel in my stomach now and then... It appeared very shortly after the latest scan, so it is probably nothing, but it spins around in my mind anyway. It is getting closer to my next check up, too. Only a month until a new scan, I have them every third month. Still nothing from the doctor in Sweden...

It took a while before I gave anyone the address of my website. I don't know what I was afraid of, and I didn't really know where I was going with it. What I know for sure is that it had a very good mental effect of writing down some of what I was thinking about.

Tuesday 21 October 2008

Finally I received a reply from Sweden! The answer was that I may come when I want, so we head down either next weekend or the first weekend in November. I just have to clarify some accommodation and someone to look after the children first. I don't have very high hopes about this, but I hope to learn a little about how they do this in Sweden, and maybe about the Swedes' attitudes regarding gene therapy in China.

Today I played "Truth or nut" with the kids. I asked my daughter if she had ever lied to me. She got a bit embarrassed and admitted that she had lied to me once. I had to ask when, and she told me that, believe it or not, she had eaten snow, a long time ago, even though she was not allowed! Well, something tells me that I just have to enjoy this age of my children.

How important our children are and have been to me these years is not possible to describe with words! I love them more than anything else on this earth, and for them I will fight the cancer until the end!

Friday 24 October 2008

Now I've just returned home from a school trip, into the wood, with my son's class. For the first time I'm actually a little happy that I have the opportunity to stay home. He is really struggling at school during the day and every day it is a fight to get him there. I must take him there (we live about 500 mtr away), drop in during their breaks and then go and get him at the end of the day. He blames it on being afraid of some bigger boys, but there may be many things that cause his fear. The teacher is sick so they must have a substitute, there are rumors that the school is going to be closed and the children moved to another school and at last (but probably not least) he knows that I'm sick and he wants to be with me most of the time... Though I really do not think the latter is the reason either. He has known about me and the illness for a long time, and the few times it has bothered him, he has been very clever to ask what happens.

Sometimes I feel degraded to be a full-time housewife. It has been the consequence of quitting my job and staying at home. The strange thing is that the transition from being a full time career woman and staying at home is not as big as I would have believed. I don't get to do more at home, either. It just takes longer time. But I do get to spend a lot more time with the children. I think that is a good thing. But what if they get even more dependent on me and something happens? Hmm, I probably have too much time to think...

I wonder what it's like to grow up with a sick mother? I

remember when we told the kids how serious my diagnosis was when I got metastases. First, we chose not to say anything. We only told them that I was sick again, but nothing about how serious it was. This bothered me a lot. I felt that I lied to them, that I was not honest with them. At the time when I got the first recurrence and the prognosis was so critical, the kids were 4 and 6 years old. How do you tell them that their Mom is going to die? After a while, a couple of months, my daughter began to ask me questions about the cancer, and I decided it was time to let her know. She was, of course, very sad. I don't believe she understood everything, but she kept asking more questions and finally then, she had the full picture. Her first reaction was quite spontaneous, "Have you told this to Dad?" and the next was whether her little brother was informed. He was not, so her instructions were very clear: he should be told as soon as possible! The worst thing was not how bad it was, but that they were not informed! And in retrospect, I must agree with her, to be held outside is not good in any context! My son's reply, after we told him, was, "ok, what's for dinner?"

Monday 27 October 2008

Sometimes I feel that I must use considerable persuasive skills to convince others that I actually feel good, both physically and psychologically. At least in relation to the cancer...

Right now I'm sitting with a lump in my throat again after fighting to get my son to go to school. I do not understand what's wrong. During the weekend he was fine, but this morning he was sick and had a stomachache again. Fortunately, a good substitute for the day was very understanding, so she told him that she would follow him *all the time during the day, even during breaks. It seemed like that eased things a bit for him, and the mom went home crying of gratitude...*

I have received a message from my sister on the blog page. Terrific! A slightly strange way to communicate, but nice! I feel that the feedback makes me stronger, I have an inner strength and others are able to see it! (Even in China) Thank you, dear sister! I love you, too!

It appears that my son struggled more with the situation than his sister, after all. It is a good thing to have people around us to lean on in these situations!

Thursday 30 October 2008

Today it was confirmed that people say a lot of crap in order to be nice. I took my son to school today, without makeup and I hadn't even combed my hair. Yet there was another mother who says I look so great! Of course it's nice to hear you look great, but today it was not true! I feel like crap, and look like it too!

Sunday 2 November 2008

Whew! Finally, it is Sunday night! What a weekend: Halloween, three (!) birthdays and family dinner. Very nice, but now I'm very tired... Last night we celebrated my father-in-law's birthday, and we left the kids with my parents-in-law for the night. So today, my husband and I have been out with the boat, alone. It was great, really nice weather, but maybe a little bit cold, we even had to break the ice on the water in some places. The downside to having a day without the kids is that you get a lot of time on your own... Both to think and feel.

Tomorrow I'll call the hospital and ask if they can check my stomach with ultrasound, I am afraid there is something wrong and I don't want to wait until December and my regular check up! Luckily, I have a very nice doctor at the local hospital. I can call him anytime and get an appointment whenever I want.

Finally I received a confirmation from the physician in Gothenburg. He writes that he is probably not more competent than the doctors I am seeing in Norway, but that it's always ok to get a second opinion and it might be nice to talk to someone else with experience with this cancer. He seems very straightforward.

Monday 3 November 2008

After taking my son to school today I got really depressed over him struggling so much, and I was also afraid there was something going on in my stomach. On the way home from school, I walked with tears in my eyes, so when I was invited in for coffee at one of my best friend and neighbour's house, the tears started flowing. Today it was really great to have someone to talk to!

When I got home I got the hospital on the phone, and I got to come in there right away. After a couple of minutes with the ultrasound he confirmed there was nothing bad going on. What a relief! At least one thing less to be concerned about...

To be surrounded by friends and positive people is invaluable to anyone, but when you really get to test yourself in life, you learn how important they really are!

Friday 7 November 2008

We finally went to see the Swedish doctor. We were greeted by the doctor at Sahlgrenska, as agreed. He was very nice. I felt that he was more optimistic than the doctors I've talked to at home. Among other things, he was very positive about the fact that it seems like my tumor isn't as fast growing as it might be for this kind of tumor. The Swedish doctor was very focused on detecting new metastases as soon as possible. He had some specific suggestions, which I will discuss with my doctors when I see them next time, regarding scanning and detecting metastases at an earlier stage. They do a scan called octreotide scintigraphy, a scan with a radioactive injection responding to the neuroendocrine cells. He also received a copy of my medical record and should discuss it with a colleague who works with this cell type. He will check out if there are any studies going on in preventive medication and if there are any documented effect of gene therapy in China. He smiled a bit when we talked about the last, but he didn't dismiss it in the same way as the Norwegian doctors have done. Han promised to send me a letter within two weeks.

Some people make a stronger impression on you than others. The doctor in Sweden made a huge impression on me. He didn't need to take time for me at all, but several times he has answered my emails and the way he greeted me was awesome. He took off his own time to meet me. If only everyone knew how important this courtesy is. Feeling that you matter, that you are important!

Regarding the gene therapy, both the Norwegian and Swedish doctors have dismissed it as not possible, but we have now, in fact, two positive cases in our Facebook group.

Monday 10 November 2008

I just hate Mondays! Today has been crazy. Before two o'clock, I had been at school four (!) times. First to deliver (which by the way went bad), then to check that all went well and finally to get both kids that finished at different times. And the house is a mess. Right now I don't feel that the world is going my way... Friday afternoon I called the Norwegian Radium Hospital and asked to get the kind of scan that they use in Sweden, but the doctor hadn't heard of it before! And I was told that I had to realize that not everything was done in the same way everywhere and that the Norwegian Radium Hospital has much better doctors than other places, and they are a lot better at interpreting the images captured... And as if that wasn't enough, I called them seven weeks ago and asked for answers as to whether they had or hadn't removed both my ovaries, because that is what the chief doctor there blurted out the last time I was there. "My doctor" says that of course they had, but she promised to check it up anyway, and when I called last Friday she told me that the pathalogs only have found one. "But," she said, "It doesn't matter, because you will have to have surgery again soon and we can remove the other then!" I am considering strongly immigrating to Sweden, where there right now is a nice, dedicated specialist who helps me on his own free time!

My ovaries. Actually, I feel sometimes that I could write a whole book about them....

As it turned out that the metastases was in my ovaries instead of my lymphs, it was possible to operate. The first time I was operated on for the tumor in the cervix, doctors decided to remove the uterus and cervix. The ovaries, they decided to leave, because I was so young. Removing them would start menopause too early, and they considered it *unfortunately because, among others, the risk of osteoporosis. Besides, the doctor said, they had never experienced before, that this kind of cancer had spread to the ovaries....But it did! When it finally was confirmed that the metastases was in fact in the ovary, it was decided to remove them both. It was done, or in retrospect, we could say they tried to have it done. I had a tumor in the right ovary, which was removed. The following year I got a cyst on the left (Which was supposed to have been removed as well). The removal of my left ovary was again attempted along with the cyst. And again I thought that now it was certainly gone. But it was only until the superior doctor who read through my journal incidentally asked me why I had not removed it (asked me!).... Pathology reports say that, in fact, only one is removed! Ergo, I still have one left.*

Wednesday 12 November 2008

Life goes up and down. Today I had a very good day. First, lunch and girl talk with my best friend. It's amazing how good it feels to get a good talk.

Afterwards, both the kids brought friends home for dinner. In the end we were 8 for dinner instead of four. I love it when we are so many, and I love to have the energy to serve them all!

Now I'm packed and ready to go on a two-day tax seminar with my old work and other similar offices in our county. It will be nice to get an update on my working skills and to see old colleagues again. Not that I am planning on going back to work again soon, but it is always ok to be updated. In order to cover the cost I have promised to give a speech about the future of the accounting business.

My sister told me today that she learns more about how I am doing when she reads my posts here, than when she is talking to me, and it's probably true. Here I can tell about anything without risking getting questioned or pitied. On the other hand, I have probably not been as emotionally unstable before, as I have been the last few weeks. Now I am happy that I'm going away for a couple of days, because I believe that sitting at home, alone most of the time, doesn't bring much good. It is probably not only the extra weight on my ass that makes it difficult to get up off the couch.

Having to quit my job was hard. I had started a new job only a year and a half before I got sick the first time. A job with many challenges, but with plenty of great colleagues and experiences. After working as an auditor for several years, I had decided to accept a job offer as manager of an accounting company. A well renowned company with about fifteen employees. I loved my new job, to be a leader and the contact with the clients. I felt that I could give more to my clients in my new job, than I could as an auditor. This was probably also the reason I was so eager to get back to work after I was sick the first time. There was plenty to deal with the period when I was back at work, and one of the great things that happened was the decision to move office to new premises. First day on the job in the brand new office, I got the phone call from my doctor that the cancer had metastasized....

Monday 17 November 2008

Who am I really trying to fool? Well it is probably myself, when I go on a two-day tax seminar. The probability of ever going to need these skills is actually minimal. Anyway, it was very nice to see old colleagues again. I even believe some of them thought it was nice to see me again, as one of them said, "damn, there is life in you!" I should perhaps have been better at visiting the office once in a while.

I know that I am no longer able to stay as focused as I used to. Chemo brain, I guess. When I was giving my speech I lost focus several times, suddenly I just forgot what I was talking about and started stuttering. I concluded by excusing myself for being a bit unfocused, but I have never heard such a great response to such an excuse. Virtually all muttered "Oh no, we didn't notice anything" in unison. Those who didn't were newly employed and didn't know my story. Sometimes it's nice to get some understanding.

Tuesday 25 November 2008

It doesn't happen too much these days, but I feel good, so I shouldn't complain... Today I took my son into town. First I saw an orthopedic surgeon to get some special fitted shoes for my swollen lymphedema leg, then we went to the school nurse at the local health center to talk about his problems at school. They are going to help us. First a psychologist will be in contact with school to get an arrangement that makes him a little safer. I hope this will work. Although, when we were sitting there, it felt more like I had problems than my son. He was talking and joking and didn't seem to be afraid of anything. I haven't heard anything from the doctor in Sweden yet. I'll send an email and ask when to expect a letter.

Monday 1 December 2008

My husband is away on work for few days, so now the kids and I are going to enjoy ourselves, alone at home. We started the day with a lot of fighting and shouting, so we had a nice start! I confronted both of the kids and told them that we had to be nice to each other and learn to be polite. I wasn't even finishing the speech before I had to give the youngest one a timeout...

Now I am heading to a board meeting. It's nice to have something else to think about.

The accounting office I worked with participates in a chain of offices. After I became ill and had stopped working, I was asked to be on the board in the chain company. It has been great to be involved in the development of the chain, and to still be able to use some of my skills. It is also nice to think about something else than kids and housework...

Wednesday 3 December 2008

Today I have got a CT. It is a bit strange to go to the hospital, to get checked up for a rare cancer with a bad prognosis, and listen to the Minister of Health on the radio, saying that new and expensive technology should not be used for cancer patients with a poor prognosis! I wonder what he would have said if his daughter was sick!

I still have not received the letter from the doctor in Sweden, so I feel I have too little information to go on yet, but I'll find out more about what this means to me. The kids and I are alone at home a few days. We enjoy ourselves and have a good time. The house is neat and clean, so I relax all the time. Last night we tidied up a bit before the cleaning help arrived this morning. So we danced around, picking up stuff and singing, "If you see some mess, pick it up!" Suddenly I ran into my son, and he started to sing, "If you see a Mom, you give her a hug!" Then he stretched his arms up and gave me a hug. Hmmm, good kids! What would I *have done without them!*

Thursday 4 December 2008

Today the kids and I were invited for dinner at a friend of mine. It was very nice, as usual! One should be more clever to take time to meet like that in the middle of the week. Everyone must have food, and whether you make dinner for four or seven doesn't really matter. I promise that I will be better to ask people over, even in the middle of the week, or perhaps especially in the middle of the week. Tomorrow I'm going to the funeral of a friend from high school. It is sad when a young man doesn't see any other option than to take his own life. Why is it like that? Why is it someone can't find the way out of their problems? Now there is certainly no going back... I hope he has found peace now.

Thursday 11 December 2008

I've forgotten to write for some days. It is probably because I have had a lot to do and because my sister is visiting. I'm now waiting for the phone call from the hospital to know how the CT I took last week is.

The memorial service on Friday was nice. Even though the circumstances were tragic, the memorial was calm and worthy. It focused on all his nice sides and all the good memories. I found myself thinking about my situation during it all, and how unfair it is that someone doesn't want to live, while others are fighting for their lives. And then I thought maybe we could exchange... a life for another. But then I thought that if I could choose to die young, and get to be an angel that would get to see my children again sometime, or get old and not get the chance, I think in fact that I'm willing to take the risk of dying young! It sounds absolutely crazy for sure. I've got way too much time to think.

Friday 12 December 2008

Yesterday I was told that my CT was good, no sign of cancer! I'm still going in for a check up on Monday, but it is unlikely that they will find something else then. This time I got CT of both lungs and pelvis, in addition to the stomach.

I have all the time, after I became ill, been in for checkups at the Norwegian Radium Hospital every 3 months. Then I'm in one day for CT or MRI, and then back to talk to a doctor 3-4 days afterwards. These days in between are unbearable. To go and wait for the results. Have they found anything or not?

Sunday 4 January 2009

Happy New Year! It has been a long time since I wrote anything. It has been busy with Christmas and with the kids having time off from school. Now, I've just sent husband and kids to go skating so I could get a little rest and quietness on my own. I went to the hospital the Monday after I wrote last time, and as expected, there was no evidence of metastases - thankfully! The day after I got a letter from the Swedish doctor, it was actually a little disappointing. He had written very little or nothing about the alternative treatments that I had asked about. He wrote a little about the diagnostic method they used, which I have forwarded to my Norwegian doctors. They have promised to consider the scintigraphy scanning when they get more information. The amazing thing is that the doctor in Sweden sent a long article from a Norwegian doctor about the procedure!

Christmas in general has been quiet, we have been with the family and it was extra nice to gather all the family on my mother's side at one of my aunt's. We were then told that one of my cousins, who is as old as I, also has cervical cancer, but fortunately not the same cell type as mine. She had laser surgery, and has been declared cancer free. It is difficult to explain how my disease is so different. My aunt said that she thought it was nice that I had been healed (she had heard that my scan was fine), then it is not easy to explain that it is only temporary and that the doctors actually almost have given up on me!

The New Year weekend we spent up in the mountains with friends. The others went skiing, and I rested and read a book.

Because of the risk of metastases it is the normal procedure to remove some lymph nodes near the cervix once you're operated on. In my case they took many, which has led my lymphatic system to no longer work as it should. This, in turn, has led to the lymph fluid in my left leg not draining and my leg is constantly swollen. I have lymphedema in the leg.

Wednesday, 7 January 2009

I spent the entire morning reading newspapers, watching TV and sitting by the computer - and yet I have not written anything here! Fortunately, I'm not depressed, just lazy and apathetic... I haven't had a car to drive with the last days and when I'm not able to go anywhere, it feels like I'm in prison. But today I bought a new car, so now I am free to go around as I like again.

Thursday 8 January 2009

I have heard that people are afraid of talking to me, they are afraid to say something wrong. So just for the record, don't be afraid to talk to me when you meet me. You do not need to think about my illness, I am like everyone else. First and foremost, a mum and wife and I have all the same everyday problems as everyone else. I don't go around and think: I've got cancer. Rather, what to have for dinner and whether the kids rain clothes still fit. I must admit that it sometimes is a bit difficult to meet people I don't have much contact with, as one might naturally ask how you're doing. But in the queue at the supermarket or when you meet someone on the street it is not ideal to roll out the entire story, so sometimes I have said that I'm just fine, without telling about the cancer. Sometimes this can be at bit weird, especially when I hear that they have talked to someone else who knows and I pretend that everything is ok. Even though not every situation is ideal for any elaboration, I've tried to be honest and open and talk about how things are with me. So if you're one of those that I have met when I have pretended everything is ok, this is the reason. I'm probably the only one who understands what I'm trying to say here, but it doesn't matter, because this is something that has bothered me a lot and now I've at least got it out! I don't know what's worse, to blow out the whole story right in the face of completely unprepared people or to "lie" and say that everything is good...

What to say or not to say to people around me has been difficult at times. My experience with blogging is that people no longer need to ask me how I am doing, because now, they can read all about it on the internet. The strange thing is that I can notice the reduction in attention, and I kind of miss it... You get used to the attention!

Tuesday 13 January 2009

Now I had a terrible weekend! It feels like I have been arguing with everyone at home, I feel tired and alone with my problems. The worst is the fact that I felt so horribly depressed (and I don't like to be depressed, so I never am). The only thing going on in my head was that I don't want to feel this way, because I have such a short time... and this just made me more angry because the others couldn't understand the way I feel. It's not exactly an argument you throw a six or eight year old. In the midst of it all, my son yelled at me, told me how selfish I was, that there are actually other things that live in our house too! One of the Christmas hyacinths that had begun to fade - and it was our fault because we hadn't given them enough water! He was genuinely upset because of these flowers, so now I do not know when I will get to throw them in the trash...

I have been swimming today, and it was really nice! I had a great day! I just wanted to sing when I swam. And when it got a lot of people in the pool, I wanted to yell out: "What a beautiful day!" Yesterday I was not so happy. I just wanted to just swim under water. But then came an elderly man, who usually swims at the same time as me, and when I said hello and smiled at him I felt it loosen up. It felt like the smile made the tight mask in my face melt. And I was myself again! Fortunately, because on Sunday evening and Monday morning I felt like I was balancing on the edge of a big depression hole.

I am actually surprised myself, how little depression I have felt throughout this journey. Therefore, when I have felt really down, I have gotten so scared. I feel that my optimism and happy attitude to life is what actually has brought me this far. I truly believe positive thinking may play a big part in getting healed.

Friday 16 January 2009

I feel great again. Now I'm having lunch guests, actually my aunt and uncle are bringing lunch. The entire time I've been sick I have had the great benefit of my aunt's support. She has been coming to see me almost every day and helped me with whatever I needed help with. Most important is, perhaps, that she has kept coming and just been there for me. We have had countless lunches together and talked about everything. She looked after the kids when my husband picked me up in the hospital after my first chemotherapy, and the sight of me, when I got home set deep tracks in her. She told me afterwards that she went home and cried, and said she wished there was something she could do for me. She could have changed with me, she said, if she just could have stopped me from being so sick. (I looked really bad. I couldn't even recognize my own face in the mirror, large round face, seemed like no muscles were in function, big, blank eyes and completely gray.)

Unfortunately my aunt got lung cancer only a couple of years later, and passed away even before she got started on chemotherapy. She has been absolutely invaluable to me these past years, and I miss her very much!

Monday 19th January 2009

It has been a great weekend. I feel relaxed and have enjoyed myself with the children. I see that when I write here, I am more open and honest than I can be with anyone. It's a bit strange, but it feels sometimes as if I am writing in my diary in my drawer. Though I don't anymore... I choose to write this blog because - no, I really don't know. Perhaps I'm trying to be heard! Perhaps some reader can help. Or maybe I just want to be seen... I can't just write my own obituary, but this way at least I can leave a trace of my life and my thoughts. Immediately after I got the "death sentence" two years ago, I actually wrote to Oprah, hoping to be on TV in the U.S., so that someone who had a cure for me could come to my rescue. But I never heard back from her.

My sister tried to get us on another TV show home in Norway, so that we could win a trip to Euro Disney, before I got too ill to travel. But the show got closed down, and we went to Euro Disney on our own. Sometimes I just want to cry out, "Look at me! Look what can happen to any one of us! Life is unfair, can someone do something for me?" At the same time, I want to shout, "Look at me! How well you may be, even when life is a hell!" Maybe I can help someone who comes in my situation to actually turn their situation into something positive. I think in fact that I have managed that, at least in the short term.

Positive thoughts are essential! I actually found a research paper the other day that said that good quality of life and positivity has a positive impact on the prognosis of cancer. Pretty amazing, but I think it's true. Without hope - what do you have? Therefore, I think it was wrong of the doctor to say that I had no chance of surviving. There is always hope! I am the proof.

Tuesday 20 January 2009

Today I have been at a meeting at school regarding my son. Happily, things have gotten a bit better lately, so things tend to ease up on their own. Anyway, the school nurse has been having conversations with him, and I don't know whether to laugh or cry over her response. Like we have thought he has been quite concerned about me. He knows that the cancer is dangerous and that I can die of it. And then he wondered what happens if both his parents die? What about the children? Well, he thought, maybe we had some friends they could live with, if not he could sit in the local grocery store with a poster around his neck saying, "one dollar" - because it was not too expensive, maybe someone could afford to buy him... Today I built Legos with him, made pancakes and read a bit extra on the bedside...

This has actually been one of my toughest experiences, and put things in perspective. I've never really been afraid of dying, but dying from... The fact that your kid is thinking about and worrying about how to get on with their life if or when you die is unbearable. It's just so unfair that we should have to put the kids through this!

When you spend a lot of time alone in a hospital, you have plenty of time to think. I remember thinking a lot about how my husband was going to cope being alone with the children. I didn't worry about how he would manage to take care of the kids alone. I felt pretty confident that he would manage that part. But the drain in the bathroom! How would he manage to clean it up? That was the first thing I showed him when I got home, totally out of perspective. Maybe it was the anesthetic...

And then I started to save money to pay for my own funeral. I also wondered if I should stop by the funeral home and plan the ceremony. But since I knew the woman that worked there, I knew that I would start crying when I talked to her, so I decided to wait a while... The money I *saved for my funeral we have spent on holidays.*

While writing this, it has been four years since my last metastases. I have been living with the cancer hanging over my head for seven and a half years. I am sick of it, and I won't do it anymore. I have decided to consider myself as cured. I live my life as if I am going to survive the cancer. I am planning on getting old.

Debbie is one of our longtime sisters that came to us from Cancer Comrades. She is in Canada and has been a rock of strength and wisdom. We are so fortunate to have her in our sisterhood.

Debbie's story:

So I've been asked to write a story about how I ended up being a proud member of the SCCC sister group. My story is not unique, in fact, it is quite similar to the other girls, located all around the world. In October 2007, two weeks after my father had passed away, I went to my very first Ob/Gyn appointment. This was after many months of persuading my family doctor that there was more going on than just normal excessive menstrual cycles. My Ob/Gyn did many tests, including pap smears and blood tests, and concluded that everything was normal. At this point I was prescribed medication in order to stop the bleeding. I followed her instructions. After all, what could possibly be wrong? I had two normal pregnancies with my now teenaged children.

In January of 2008, the medication has stopped working.

After much persuasion, the Ob/Gyn reluctantly agreed to give me a partial hysterectomy. Everything returned to normal until August 2008, at which time the heavy bleeding had returned. The only explanation I was given was, "Some women, it just takes longer for their bodies to recuperate." And once again, I was prescribed more medication. In October of 2008, I ended up in the Emergency Room as the pills, again, failed to work. The on-duty doctors did a complete physical exam, and said I was probably just fatigued and that I should go back and visit my regular Ob/Gyn. In November, I went back to my Ob/Gyn, and she reluctantly agreed to remove my cervix and remaining ovary, cautioning me that it would put me into radical menopause and she did not recommend this surgery. Between November 2008, and March 2009, I had canceled the surgery appointment 3 times, as something "more important" had always come up.

March 14th 2009, I finally had my surgery, but had a very difficult time recovering. On April 2nd 2009, I heard the words that I will never forget. The doctor sat across from me at her desk and proceeded to say, "You have Small Cell Carcinoma of the Cervix." I knew the word carcinoma meant cancer, but I had never heard of small cell of the cervix. My world was spinning out of control before my eyes. I asked her to write it down, as I was alone in her office, feeling like I was going to suffocate. There was no air left in the room. I ran from her office feeling like I was suffocating and thinking to myself, "How am I going to drive home?" The last thing I remember the doctor saying to me was, "Don't go home and Google this." After hearing those words and the doctor telling me not to do any research on the cancer, I knew my world was about to change forever. I was told that in 4 days, I was to begin chemotherapy and that it was going to be aggressive. I had several scans in those four days and the doctors believed the cancer did not originate in my cervix. After two body scans, a bone scan, a brain scan and several chest scans, it was clear that the cancer had, if fact, originated in my cervix. My oncologist who has been practicing for 22 years had never had a case of SCCC. I was told if I did not start chemo, I would have approximately 6-10 weeks to live, as this cancer was extremely aggressive. Not doing chemo didn't even cross my mind. After all, I had two teenagers, stepchildren and a husband that all relied on me. I vowed to myself that I was not going to stay in bed, and that I was not going to be sick during the chemo treatments.

Many doctors at the cancer center studied my case and poked and prodded me. One radiation oncologist got my permission to write a paper about me. In this large cancer center I was the only patient the center had ever treated with small cell. I remember, at each appointment, I felt like the doctors were looking at me with sympathy in their eyes. I started a regime of 18 cycles of Etopocide and Cisplatin. Each time the burning sensation went through my arm, from the chemo running through my veins, all I could think about was my family. Although I begged the doctors to insert a port, as the pain in my veins was unbearable at times, they did not feel this was necessary. There was no way I could not take this; I had to be strong for them.

During this time my family went through Hell, my husband started drinking heavily and my kids starting acting way out of character. We sought help through a hospital therapist. After all, we had never experienced these crazy emotions. I remember one visit from my mother shortly *after I had lost my hair. She bought me a wig, as she could not stand to see me bald. My mom and my sister would regularly come and visit for short periods of time. I truly believe they could not stand to see me. My kids were wonderful, accompanying me to appointments and sitting with me through chemo. My husband was amazing, taking me to appointments, sitting with me for hours during chemo, getting me warm blankets and just looking after me.*

The chemo was very hard on my body. My white blood count would never be high enough after treatments to start the next round and, as a result, I was given daily Neupogen shots by my husband. This shot made me feel like I always had the flu. After many trips to the hospital and 7 grueling months later, chemo finally finished. After chemo, I began 42 radiation treatments, which resulted in me getting sicker and sicker by the day. Food became my enemy, but I knew I had to eat to stay strong.

During all of this, I longed for a support system. All I could find in my community was a support system for every type of cancer...except mine. I always felt alone. One night, early in my treatments, when I could not sleep, I was surfing the Internet, looking for information on SCCC. I was finding very little and very old studies with very low survival rates. Then I came across a group called Cancer Comrades. I was thrilled that there were women out there with the same type of cancer that I have. Two ladies, Melanie and Colleen, started this group with a purpose that nobody would feel alone. They tried to pair each woman up with somebody who she could easily relate to and was somewhat in proximity to where she lived. At this point, I believe there were 12 women on the site, Cancer Comrades. I spoke to my "buddy", Shawna, a few times on the phone, but sadly, the cancer had overcome her body and shortly after, she passed away. I was angry. I did not want to be around dying cancer patients. There was no way I was going to die. I became quite silent within the group during this time. A few of the original SCCC survivors were still emailing me, checking on my progress. I will never forget how excited I was when I opened their emails and read that they were, for the most part, all surviving this horrible disease. It was then brought to my attention that the group had recently opened a Facebook page for other women with the same type of cancer. I knew I just had to belong to this group so that no other woman would feel alone, as I did. I have met some amazing women along this journey, with our only commonality being SCCC. In April 2011, a few of us were able to meet in New York City for a cancer summit. Angela V. had arranged a dinner on the Thursday night. I was not going to attend, as I was afraid. These women knew my innermost secrets and I did not want to meet them in person, because it would make it real, instead of just virtual. I walked into the restaurant with my daughter and her friend and I felt like I was home. So relaxed. We chatted, laughed and cried like schoolgirls. We truly were sisters. The hugs at the end of the weekend were something I will never forget, as we had no idea if we would ever see each other again. Never knowing if the disease would take one of us. Well, the unforgettable happened to two beautiful girls that I met in NYC, Ally and Rosie. They lost their lives shortly after we met. It was very painful for me, losing Ally, as she was only 24 years old and had her whole life ahead of her. And I had met and hugged her. My pain for losing Rosie was very deep, as we were truly like sisters, spending time emailing and talking on the phone. Even though she lived in Minnesota, it often felt like she lived around the corner and we had met in person in NYC. She, too, was real.

At this point, I again reevaluated my purpose in this group. Losing girls that I had met was very painful. I wanted to leave the group and just move on with my life, as I was cancer-free now and really wanted to forget how painful my cancer treatments were. I just couldn't leave. There were more and more women joining and I had to give them some hope. I was a 16- month survivor at this point, and other girls needed to know that. I continued to support the girls where I could. I drove 4 hours in the rain, one way, to Rochester, NY, to visit a cancer sister who was losing her battle and was in the hospital. I spent a few hours with Sarah, knowing I would never see or talk to her again and not sure she knew I was even there. But I just had to go and hold her. Over the course of this journey, many women have lost their battle with SCCC and more and more are surviving. When we lose someone, I no longer want to run from the group. I motivate myself to do more in the group and raise awareness of this disease.

Our group, that was started by two ladies from the US, now has members from Norway, Australia, the UK, the US and Canada. Nineteen of us met in Las Vegas in March 2012. Again, we laughed, cried and hugged, knowing when we left that we may never see some of the girls again. But I would not trade this experience for anything. I have driven 5 hours, one way, to Michigan to spend one night with Melanie, just because we are "sisters". I truly believe if it was not for the hope and love of Melanie, Angela V., Jaclyn, Jen and Colleen, in the early days, I am not sure I would have survived. The vision of a few pioneers in this group has raised over $100,000.00 for a Small Cell Carcinoma of the Cervix research project, through MD Anderson. We *have brought awareness to this cancer and have managed to engage a "group doctor", Dr. Michael Frumovitz, who is driving our research project. He is also a member of our group and has provided valuable advice for some of our sisters. We have sold bracelets, t-shirts, magnets, made a video and have now written a book to help raise awareness and money for our research project.*

My journey has enabled me to see life from a completely different angle. In the last almost 4 years, since that frightful day, I have learned to appreciate the very small things in life.

It has now been almost 3 years since the treatments have finished, and each time I go to the doctor, I feel grateful when he says, "You are still cancer free." The last time I was there, in summer 2012, my doctor said to me, "You are a perfect example of a medical miracle and I honestly did not think you would survive."

My hope is that, with this awareness, another woman with SCCC will never feel alone. Everything in life does happen for a reason, although it may not seem like it at the time, there can be positive outcomes from the most negative situations. I will never forget those words, "The prognosis is poor, and without treatment, you will have 6 weeks to live."

My dad was my guardian angel during my journey. We were so close, I believe he lead me through.

Debbie Whyet

September 2012

Danielle Dick's Story

My story.

My name is Danielle Dick and I live in Australia. I was 23 years old, newly engaged and the director of a childcare centre when diagnosed with cancer.

In April 2011, I had a cone biopsy of my cervix performed due to some Adenocarcinoma, pre-cancerous cells being discovered. These cells were not cervical cancer, however, they had the potential to progress into cervical cancer and needed to be removed surgically. Following this procedure, I was having PAP smear tests more regularly; these tests came back negative for any cancerous cells in November 2011 and April 2012, so my gynecologist told me that he would perform another one in 12 months time, making me due for my next one in April 2013. However, in November 2012, I started to feel like something was wrong. My own intuition/gut feeling was telling me, urging me to go back and test again. So 6 months before I was due for another PAP smear, I booked in and did another one anyway.

It turns out my intuition was right. This PAP test came back abnormal with what we all thought were some more pre-cancerous cells. The gynecologist referred me to a pre-cancer specialist. The reason for this referral was that he felt that he could not remove the pre-cancerous cells again without further weakening my cervix and that the specialist may know how to remove them safely.

This specialist, Dr. Michael Campion, did another PAP test to ensure it was not a false positive reading and this is when my Hell began. I was lucky that Dr. Campion had a team of pathologists working directly for him. These pathologists do only gynecology pathology, and screening for Small Cell Carcinoma is included in all PAP tests, even though the chances of it showing on a PAP smear are minimal. When these pathologists ran my test they found what they thought was evidence of a Small Cell Neuroendocrine tumour. Dr. Campion asked me to come in for a consultation to break the news of their suspicion. This meeting was 2 days after Christmas, 27th December 2012. I was told that the situation was now potentially a whole lot worse than we had originally thought and that pre-cancerous cells were not the concern now, that a rare and aggressive tumour was now the concern. I was told not to panic, that this is so rare that the chances of it actually being a small cell tumour were very slim.

Dr. Campion informed me that there were many professionals in the gynecology industry, as well as the pathologists that tested my smear, showing interest in my case, as it was very rare for this tumour to show in a PAP test and that this could be a breakthrough. The specialist suggested that we don't talk about treatment options unless it is confirmed, as we need to cross that bridge when we come to it. However, chemotherapy was very likely should I have this tumour. I agreed with Dr. Campion and chose not to discuss treatment of a tumour that was not confirmed. I was thinking I probably didn't have it anyway.

I had emergency surgery for biopsies. A total of 7 tissue biopsies were taken, 3 from the cervix, 2 from the cervical canal, and 2 from my uterus. 4 days after the surgery I got the devastating phone call confirming the cancer. I will never forget that moment. Sitting at my parents' house, I answered the specialist's phone call. I was expecting to be told it was not this aggressive cancer and the pathology had been wrong. I expected this because I had been told that my chances of actually having Small Cell Neuroendocrine tumours were so slim. But as I heard Dr. Campion say, "Listen Sweetheart, those biopsies have confirmed that it is neuroendocrine cancer." I lost my breath. I was asked to attend an appointment with a surgical oncologist the following week. It was almost like I was in shock, everything became cloudy and I felt like I was watching my own life through a movie. I got off the phone, my mum staring at me waiting for information, and all I could manage to say, my voice breaking and tears rolling down my cheeks was, "Mum, I have a tumour." Mum burst into tears and gave me a hug and just at that moment, my fiancé walked through the front door. I looked at him and said, "I have it; I have that tumour they thought." My fiancé had been to all my appointments previously and knew the exact information I did, so that's all the explanation he needed. That afternoon I was in for a CT scan to ensure the small cell cancer was only present in my cervix and had not metastasized to other organs.

I met with the surgeon the following week and was completely shattered when she told me that a radical hysterectomy was the best course of action. I could not believe what I was hearing. I am the director of a childcare centre as a profession and I had built my life around children. To lose the ability to carry a child was the single most devastating part of this entire cancer journey. The remainder of that appointment is like a foggy memory. I barely remember what was said and I am thankful that my family attended with me to ask all of the questions I could not, including the possibility of harvesting my eggs.

It was this night that I found The Sisterhood. I remember

being so quiet, surrounded by family but not being able to say a word. I was like a zombie. And my sister and I were sitting next to each other, researching the cancer, trying to find something that would give us some hope. My sister came across a forum called "team inspire," which was where lots of SCCC sisters met before the Facebook page was established. On this forum was a link to the Facebook page. It felt so good to know that there were other women out there who had been through this horrible experience, and I could somehow contact them.

The radical hysterectomy was performed 6 days later, with the removal of my cervix, uterus and 24 pelvic lymph nodes. A fertility doctor was also present at the surgery to examine my ovaries. They decided to leave both ovaries and remove a piece of the left ovary for freezing. They intended to re-implant this part of my ovary in my arm, should my ovaries be irreversibly damaged by chemotherapy.

The pathology reports from the radical hysterectomy (RH) showed the Small Cell Neuroendocrine tumour was 12mm by 11mm, no larger than the size of a jellybean. 1 lymph node out of the 24 removed and tested was infected with small cell cancer. However, this lymph node contained only a 2mm tumour, it did not look irregular and the doctors and pathologists were confident that this was the very first spread of the cancer and it had been caught in its very early stages. They called this a micro metastasis. I am so lucky I had this caught so early.

2 days after the RH and during my hospital stay, I began fertility injections to prepare my eggs for harvesting. These injections were daily for 14 days and then another day surgery to collect the eggs. These eggs were then fertilized by my fiancé and 3 surviving embryos have been frozen for surrogacy options later.

I started chemotherapy 2 days after the egg collection, a mixture of Carboplatin and Etoposide, 3 consecutive days, 21 days apart. I have a total of 6 rounds.

You hear many horror stories about chemotherapy, however, I have coped with it quite well. There are many side effects from these drugs, but it's amazing how my body just did what it had to and coped with it the best it could. Side effects included: hair loss, nausea, sensitive teeth, pimples, aching muscles, gritty eyes, mouth ulcers, headaches and weight loss. Hair loss was probably one of the hardest side effects to endure as a woman. I found it hard to feel like a woman after losing my uterus and my hair, but it's true what they say, it grows back so quickly. As I write this story I am on my 5th round of chemotherapy with my 6th and final next week, and my hair has begun growing back in between these rounds. I don't know if it will fall out again after next week, but at least I now know how quickly it grows back when the chemotherapy leaves my system.

We have met with the surgical oncologist, chemotherapist and radiation oncologist at the cancer centre where I have my treatment, to discuss the need for radiation to the pelvis following chemo. We have all decided that it is not necessary in my case and I will not be having it. The reason for this decision is that the doctors are VERY confident all the cancer was removed during the RH. Chemotherapy was a precaution in case any rogue cancer cells may be floating around my body looking for a home. The chemo will kill these. Radiation is another precaution, there is always the possibility that some residual cancer cells are lurking in the pelvis, however, the chemotherapy would already be assisting with killing these if they were present. After long discussions and my medical team seeking advice from many professionals both in Australia and overseas, they told me that there was no evidence for them to recommend radiation for me. That there was nothing to say it would be of benefit.

Also, I was told by my medical team that small cell tumours USUALLY (and I stress the word usually because there are sisters out there who have proved this wrong) does not reoccur in the pelvis. It is a nasty beast that would normally invade the bloodstream or lymphatic system and find a new home in another organ, totally unrelated to the pelvis area. By choosing to have radiation I would only be lowering my risk of the cancer returning in the pelvis, not anywhere else. And I would be doing this with the risks of permanent damage being done to my bowel, bladder and other internal organs. Also the short time side effects are something I needed to consider also, such as diarrhea, radiation burns, stenosis, etc.

So the decision has been made to complete the chemotherapy and not have radiation. I am confident that I left no stone unturned, I did lots of research about the best ways to beat this cancer, as did my medical team. I am confident in the treatment course I am having.

The sisterhood has been absolutely amazing throughout this experience. It's amazing how lonely you can feel through treatment. I felt like I had so much love and support around me from my family, but at the same time, none of them had to do what I did, none of my family had to feel the way I was, and that just feels so lonely and terrifying. To find a group of women who know how that feels, who have all had to have treatment for the same thing and who are there to answer all your questions and concerns is truly amazing.

The sisterhood is so supportive, they give words of encouragement when needed, they give advice, they give hope and they pass on all their love. It's like having a family with some members I have never met, yet we all feel so close to one another. The sisterhood gave me hope when I felt I had none.

I am now concentrating on my attitude towards this cancer. I was so full of anger and hurt and confusion about it all that I lost focus of what truly mattered. I lost focus on the fact that I'm alive, I had this cancer caught early, and there is hope that I will live for a long time yet. I heard someone say, "If it weren't for cancer I would have the perfect life... but if it weren't for cancer I would not know it." This is so true. Cancer has opened my eyes to the world and made me appreciate each day as it comes. I am going to stay positive that I can beat this, and with the support of fellow sisters fighting the same disease, we will get through these tough times.

Sasha Brotto's Story:

August 18th, 2008 is a day I will never forget. A day that will forever be burned into my mind. The day I first heard the words, "Sasha, it's cancer." At the time it felt so surreal and all I could think about was that I was going to be late to pick the boys up from school. At the time I was a 31 year-old, single mum with three beautiful boys, Samuele (7),

Sebastian (5) and Stefano (2).

I had gone to see my GP after I had noticed and felt something that didn't seem right. I also had irregular bleeding. My GP suggested a PAP test and the results of this test showed abnormal cells. I was diagnosed with cancer.

I sat there in complete disbelief and thought to myself it had to be a mistake, I felt fine and I didn't have time to be sick. I needed to be a mother and I had things to do. I remember watching my Nonna and my Godmother on their cancer journeys and I thought to myself, "It won't be that bad. I'm young and it might still be an easy fix." It wasn't until I was sitting in my car, waiting to pick my son up from school and talking to a friend on the phone, that it really sunk in. I was going to be sick.

What followed from that moment changed not only my life, but the lives of my 3 boys, my family and my friends. Telling the people I loved the most was one of the hardest things I have ever had to do. How do you tell your parents something like this and, even worse, how do you tell your beautiful young children? No parents ever want to hear that their child is sick and no children ever want to hear that their mum is sick. I remember looking at my boys that night and giving them the biggest hugs. They've had enough to deal with already. How was this going to affect them?

I required a colposcopy with biopsies and so, a few days later, I had my first appointment with my gynecologist. The end result of my appointment was that things didn't look good. All I wanted to know was what was going to happen next? The gynecologist referred me to another specialist, Deb, who I ended up seeing the following week. I had questions but words escaped me and, if you know me, you know that this doesn't happen often.

Deb had a look at my cancer and brought it up on the screen for my sister and me to see. I looked directly at it and said to myself, "Leave me alone, GO AWAY, I don't want or need you in my body." I will never forget what it looked like. I was told that it was a rare form of small cell cancer called Adenocarcinoma Small Cell Neuroendocrine, which is normally only found in the brain or lung.

That night I told my boys about what was happening. I explained that Mummy is sick and that the doctors are going to do everything they can to make me better. I told them that I would get sick from the medicine and that I would lose my hair. Stefano gave me a hug and Sebastian asked if he could leave the room to play the Wii. Samuele said, "Wait here," and he ran to get some paper and a pen. When he came back he drew a picture and said, "Mum you have to stay like this /\/\/\/\/\ not this -------------." Just like in the movies. I promised to do my best!

I was then referred to Peter Mac Hospital and not long after that I started my first round of chemo. Over the next 4 months I endured 5 rounds of chemo, each one lasting for three days, as well as 42 fractions of external pelvic radiation (1 per day) and 4 internal radiations. I spent most of this time in the hospital, away from my kids, my family and my friends. I was in extreme pain and was fighting for my life. I was sick on a daily basis, had absolutely no appetite and barely had the energy to function.

My treatment finished in December, just before Christmas, and on the 6th January 2009, I received the news that I had gone into remission. Just when I thought it was over they told me I required prophylactic whole brain radiation to prevent central nervous system metastasis from forming. This commenced in March 2009, and I had treatment on a daily basis for about a month.

Although the worst of it is over and I am almost 5 years post diagnosis, the cancer and its treatment has affected all aspects of my life. I am a completely different person now. My priorities have changed and this journey has taught me a lot about myself and the people around me.

I now look at life very differently and can always find the silver lining. It doesn't matter how bad today is, tomorrow will be a better day. I have realized that I am a lot stronger than I ever thought.

It's now 2013, and for the first time since diagnosis, I no longer feel alone. I found a group of women on Facebook with the same cancer. Just knowing there are others out there, going through what I went through, makes me feel less alone. I cannot express in words what a feeling it is. Being able to share our journeys, our ups, our downs, our fears and our triumphs creates a bond stronger than the cancer ever could. We are sisters and I am so glad to have met 5 of these special ladies recently and look forward to meeting more in the future.

I hope my story will encourage women of all ages to be aware of their bodies and to be proactive in protecting themselves and their families from this rollercoaster ride. Make sure you continue to get regular PAP tests and if you ever feel that something isn't right, speak to your doctor because you never know what is around the corner. My journey does not end here. It has taken a new path to help create awareness and, one day, I hope a cure to this "rare but there" cancer.

Tammy Jone's Story:

Hi,

My name is Tammy Jones and I am 37 years old. I live in Halifax, West Yorkshire, UK. I have 3 children, two boys aged 13 and 16 and a daughter age 3. I went for a routine smear in July 2010, thinking all would be fine as usual. That was until my doctor called me back in and explained my smear had not come back normal. She then sent me for a colposcopy so they could determine what was wrong. I wasn't too worried, as I'd been fit and healthy, had a 1 year-old daughter and was living a hectic life. Two weeks later I went back to the doctor (July 26th 2010) and was told I had cancer. I was shocked, but had a family holiday with my 3 children and 2 stepchildren booked for August, so my specialist said I was okay to go. I still wasn't having any problems on my return visit on September the 8th. That's the day my world fell apart. I had already accepted I had cancer but thought a hysterectomy would solve that. But now my specialist told me it was this rare cancer they didn't really know about and was sending me to St. James Hospital Leeds, our closest rare cancer specialized hospital. I went to see them on the 10th of September and they explained I couldn't have a hysterectomy, as my treatment had already been delayed by my previous doctor. That day was the hardest in my life. The doctors were talking but all I really heard was "poor prognosis," "don't know how to treat," and "be prepared for us to prolong not treat." I'm sure they said a lot more but, at the time, all I could think was, is this really me who can't be helped? I was healthy didn't have any problems. They told me my treatment would start 5 days later on the 15th of September. I went home to my kids and parents and told them everything. We were all distraught but also in disbelief. I trawled the Internet for hours but everything was the same. Poor prognosis. Death. That was all I could find.

I started my treatment with three 3-day cycles of Cisplatin and Etoposide every two weeks. It was awful and knocked me sick and so tired, but my kids kept me going. I lost my hair roughly 3 weeks into treatment. It was so hard when the clumps started coming away but eventually, I loved how easy it was not having hair to worry about. Then the external radiation started for 6 weeks, every day, and once a week chemo. At first it wasn't too bad but as the days wore on I became so tired and run down. At times I honestly thought, "Can I do this?" I even felt like my days were ending and had some very dark days. Because I was on steroids I also put 3 stone on in weight. The steroids played havoc with me turned me into a shaky, short-tempered, emotional wreck. The last 3 weeks of external radiation I began 3 cycles of internal radiation. The first one was awful. I cried so much and was so uncomfortable I just wanted to give in and stop everything. I felt so down, my hair was gone, I had put on so much weight and ten people were all playing about down in my most personal area. I didn't need that. I cried for days but my children soon made me realize that I felt like I did because I was getting better for them. I finished my radiation treatments on Christmas Eve and wasn't supposed to start my chemo cycles until January, so I enjoyed my family time. I then completed a further 3 cycles of chemo and in March 2011, I got the all clear. Even to this day I'm in shock. Cancer changed my life forever and I didn't believe I would get better, but then they told me I'd won the fight. I have been left with neuropathy, quite severely, from treatment. But *any physical pain is never as bad as the emotional torture I had thinking I wouldn't be here to see my children grow. I, sadly, only found the SCCC/LCCC Sisters Facebook page after treatment had finished, but I am so thankful I did. They understand how you feel when words can't explain it. They help you make sense of life and when you have no one who understands, you have these ladies to help you keep strong and even smile. I'm forever thankful for the support they all give. The friendship between people who have never met is amazing. It's these ladies who are going to help find a cure and bring people together from all over the world. Thank you, from my inside out.*

Raylee Mascord's Story:

THAT TIME I HAD CANCER by Raylee Mascord

The Christmas of 2011 will be remembered, not for the 6-hour stint on Christmas Eve, setting up a new swing-set for my then 22-month old daughter, but as one of the last days I would feel physically well for some time. And one of the last days before the life I knew previously, would be irrevocably changed.

On Christmas afternoon, my daughter developed a head cold and two days later I was showing symptoms of the same cold. The cold seemed to lift around New Year's but in the first week of January I noticed that the symptoms were lingering. In the second week of January I began to experience sharp headaches on my left temple, and a stabbing pain behind my left eye. The headaches would last *for several hours at a time, go away and then come back later in the day. After two weeks the headaches had become generalized, with pain and pressure all over my head, were excruciating, and were lasting six to eight hours each day. As I rarely experienced headaches, and they were not responding to over-the-counter treatments, after three weeks, I saw my GP. After examining me for more serious conditions and given the earlier cold, my doctor concluded that the source of the headaches was sinusitis, and suggested a combination of anti-inflammatory tablets and menthol lozenges.*

Over the next two days, the treatment worked and the sinus fluid was released down the back of my nose and throat. My throat and tongue became swollen to the point that I had difficulty speaking and eating. The next day I noticed changes in my vision. My left eye field of view appeared blurred in conditions of bright or dim light and there was sharp muscular pain on the outside of my eye whenever I moved my eyeball. The same night I noticed that my tongue and lips were numb or tingly most of the time.

The next day I felt patches of numbness and tingling in my left foot and hand. The nerve symptoms were worse at night when I was at rest. Then the numbness would slowly creep up my leg to my knee. I had involuntary movements like my whole leg twitching about a foot in the air. The most disconcerting of symptoms occurred through the night. I would wake up to the strange sensation as though my brain was rattling in my skull, other times it would feel like my eyeballs were shaking in their sockets or a feeling of an electrical buzzing between the hemispheres of my brain. Sometimes I would wake to a flashing paralysis up and down my arms and legs, extreme itchiness of facial skin, and a blurring of the vision in my left eye in dim or bright light. One night I awoke to the rattling brain sensation and had a total loss of vision in one eye. I had also lost my sense my sense of balance and veered off to one side when attempting to walk. These symptoms were frightening and I visited my GP several times in an attempt to find answers. I recall a conversation with my doctor where I explained that these were not normal sensations for me, and I believed that something was very amiss in my body, that something was out-of-control and causing the neurological symptoms. I did have a sense that it was cancer, even at this early stage, and knowing that my GP had experienced cancer himself, many years ago, I knew that he knew exactly what I was saying. I pleaded with my G.P to help me find the cause of the frightening symptoms. A CT scan and MRI of brain showed no indication of any issue that would be causing such symptoms. The neurologist I was referred to suggested that I was just experiencing depression and anxiety, which I found extremely frustrating and condescending. However, I knew my body, and my mind and was confident that the symptoms were not psychosomatic in any way, shape or form. The neurological symptoms remitted after 8 weeks, with the only sign of the experience being permanent "floaters" across my whole visual field in bright light or sunlight.

I also noticed that I was incredibly mentally fatigued at this time. I would be standing and would feel the need to sit down, and as soon as I sat, I would feel the need to lie down, and within seconds I would feel this incredible drowsiness overtake me and I would be asleep almost immediately. It was the type of sleep that it difficult to wake up from; I literally was unable to rouse myself into wakefulness for several hours. If my sleep was disturbed, I would fall immediately back into a drowsy slumber. Physical fatigue increased too. I found it incredibly challenging to keep up with my very active toddler, which I had previously enjoyed.

Approximately three weeks after the neurological symptoms began, I began to experience bleeding from my urethra. The anti-inflammatory medication that my GP had prescribed listed bleeding as a side effect, so it was discontinued, but the bleeding continued. It would start off a dark, red colour and get lighter over a couple of weeks, appear to remit, and then become dark again. As time went on, the hemorrhaging became heavier and eventually the loss of blood from my urethra was continuous. I approached my GP and several other doctors about the haematuria, but all told me that it wasn't possible for that amount of blood to be coming out of my urologic system. On a few occasions there was also a bright, red vaginal blood occurring, but as it was only on one or two days, and would usually remit quickly, and the urethral bleeding was continual, I didn't pay it much heed. After a week of bleeding, I had severe kidney-type (flank) pain. My GP tested for a urinary tract infection which came back negative. Another doctor, upon physical examination, agreed that the bleeding was indeed urethral, and not vaginal. Over the next months, the bleeding was accompanied by lower urinary pain and urinary urgency and frequency. Over the months of bleeding and pain, I began to feel a sense of hopelessness that the cause of the symptoms would be found in time.

On April 10th, Good Friday morning, I woke up with a full bladder but upon attempting to go to the toilet, found that I couldn't urinate. I tried again an hour later with the same results. Within the next hour I began to hemorrhage thick, dark blood through my urethra. It was this day that I also began to have heavy vaginal bleeding upon bowel motions. Wanting answers, and needing to pee, I decided to attend the emergency department for assistance. The nurse on duty was compassionate and patient, and after telling her my story of the past few months, filled me with confidence that answers were coming.

After managing to pee a very small amount, which was the consistency of tomato juice, I was soon moved to an emergency department bed for observation. The ER registrar took my history, checked out my scans, took some blood and concluded that things were within a normal range, although mentioning that some of my blood work was on the high end of normal. Probably anticipating the busy nature of a Friday evening, and also a public holiday, the doctor discharged me without further investigation, on the suggestion I seek a referral to a urologist for further investigation of the urethral bleeding. Upon querying why I was also now bleeding on bowel movements, she exclaimed dramatically, "I have no idea!"

When I saw the GP the next week, I sat in his waiting room moaning in pain. The pain was predominantly in my lower back and lower pelvis and was becoming unbearable. He said he had hoped the bleeding had remitted on its own. I told him that I was now bleeding heavily from the vagina on bowel movements, as well as the continuing urethral bleeding. This had been occurring for 62 days now and, at times, the bleeding occurred simultaneously with vaginal bleeding, even though there was no connection between the two areas. Suddenly I could see my doctor having a light bulb moment. He said, "I think the problem is a gynecological issue, impacting on the urological system." From my research of the past few months, I believed the most likely diagnosis would be uterine, bladder or cervical cancer that had spread, causing the bleeding in multiple areas. I thought it was most unlikely to be cervical, as I had had a clear PAP smear less than two years previously, which is the recommended time frame in Australia.

My GP wrote referrals to both a private urologist and a gynecologist, suggesting I could see the doctor for whichever appointment came up first. Upon calling for an appointment the next day, I was given an appointment seven weeks away for the urologist, but only a one week wait for the gynecologist. I felt amazing relief to know that I may soon know the cause of all the symptoms of the past 4 months.

The next week I felt much pain in my legs and groin lymph nodes, and had the unpleasant experience of my menstrual period, which surprisingly was still regular, exiting my body through my urethra. And two days before my gynecological appointment, the blood began to have an offensive odor.

At the appointment with the gynecologist, upon explaining my experiences over the past several months, the specialist was unbelieving that the bleeding and my menstrual period could be coming from my urethra. Upon physical examination, she said there was too much bleeding to be able to perform a PAP smear, but upon speculum and visual examination of my cervix she exclaimed, "Oh wait. What is...I'm sorry I have to get that out!" She then proceeded to reach her hand inside me and pull out handfuls of dark flesh. She did this several times, which was extremely painful and fear provoking. Amidst my screaming out, I asked incredulously, "What is that?" and was told it was a miscarriage. I told her a miscarriage wasn't a possibility as I was single, and there was no chance of conception since I birthed my daughter three years ago. She finally believed me, and admitted that the tissue was most probably a "growth" and that she needed to stop pulling at it as it was attached at my cervix. She had extracted a specimen jar full and wanted to send it to the lab for biopsy. I was now bleeding very heavily vaginally, so she told me I would have to be admitted to the local hospital to which she was attached, in case I continued to bleed and lost too much blood. She also decided that an examination under anesthetic would be required to assess the mass. Despite the pain, shock of realizing I had a tumor, and the now heavy vaginal bleeding, I was so thankful that the problem had finally been found. After talking to family members about the discovery, organizing care for my daughter and pet and packing a bag, my dad drove me to the hospital. It took several hours but later that night I was finally admitted. As I lay on a trolley in the emergency department room, the registrar had taken my details and history, and I was cannulated and offered pain medication, I could not believe that I was finally going to get the medical attention I'd been asking for, for so many months. I thought for sure, at any minute, a doctor would come in and tell me that they were discharging me, that the issue wasn't serious enough, or that they didn't know what they could do for me. But soon I was taken to the ward. Even though it was late, it didn't go unnoticed that I was being wheeled into the Gynecological Cancer Ward. Even so, the reality of cancer didn't really sink in. The plan was to squeeze me in at the end of the *surgical theatre day, but of course it was already late, so it was held over to the next day and I had a fairly sleepless night. The surgery team was unable to fit me in the next day or night, as I was on the Emergency List for surgery and there were higher priorities than me. So I was sent home for the weekend and told my bed would be reserved for Monday morning when I could return and would be amongst the first to have the examination under anesthetic (EUA). So I went home and tried to be normal, knowing that I most probably had a tumor growing inside me. When I returned to the hospital on Monday morning, the EUA was performed early and I returned to the ward. Afterwards, the lovely lady surgeon told me that the remaining mass appeared to be 4 cm in diameter, was cauliflower in shape, and was growing through and blocking my cervix in entirety. So, of course, I was Googling this and had come to the conclusion that I did indeed have cervical cancer. The ward obstetrician and a cancer care nurse confirmed the results of my Internet surfing the next afternoon, when the results of the specimen obtained by the private gynecologist were received. I was told the biopsy of the tumor had identified it as a malignant, squamous cell carcinoma of the cervix, and that further examination under anesthetic would be required to investigate spreading to other areas, and to stage the cancer. Even though it was the diagnosis that by that stage I was expecting, I was struck by the bleakness the obstetrician displayed, and the cancer care nurse's skin tone appeared a ghostly white when she entered the room. After all, I had always considered cervical cancer amongst the most easily cured of the cancers. The doctor and nurse seemed to display an attitude of defeat. I remember feeling a little matter-of-fact about the diagnosis, to the point that the nurse returned* alone to my room a few minutes later and asked me if I understood what I had just been told. I explained that I understood that I had cervical cancer, but that I was unable to process the news emotionally until I knew what the diagnosis meant for me, if and how far the cancer had spread, etc. The nurse was very kind and sat with me for a little while, gave me a whole bundle of information about cervical cancer and left me to absorb the information. I recall looking out the window at a beautiful sunset over the hills and wondering what all this would mean to my life, and my two-year-old daughter's life.

The next morning the fellow doctor of Gynecological Oncology discussed the diagnosis with me. He said that the treatment, which he believed would be most effective, would be a combination of chemotherapy and radiation. I was somewhat surprised. I couldn't understand why they couldn't just cut out the tumor or perform a hysterectomy to remove it. Chemotherapy and radiotherapy were for real, life-threatening cancers, weren't they??? I was discharged the next morning with appointments for another surgery and PET scan the next week to determine the extent of spread of the cancer.

When I returned for the EUA the next week, it was uneventful and I was discharged straight away without any further information. I was told that I could call the gynecological ward to talk to the Cancer Care team if I needed to talk.

A week later I received a discharge letter from the hospital in the mail. Most was information I had been previously told, but the correspondence defined the pathology of the tumor as being, " Poorly Differentiated, Small Cell

Neuroendocrine Carcinoma of the Cervix (Grade 3)." My immediate reaction was, "What on Earth is that?" My curiosity immediately got the better of me, and I went straight to Google to find out what that meant. Ten minutes later I wished I hadn't consulted Google. The information that all the articles reiterated was, "rare, and aggressive," "poor-prognosis," "20% survival rate," "early metastases," "average survival time of 16 months after diagnosis." I was feeling very confused and scared. Finally, after a week had passed, I called the Cancer Care team on the ward and the coordinator asked me to come in that afternoon to discuss the diagnosis. I went in, supported by my mother and sister, and had many questions prepared to ask and was expecting to hear the worst. What I was told by the doctor surprised me, and gave me hope again. He said, "Yes, it is a rare and aggressive cancer, but we think we have caught it early. We think we can cure this." When pressed, he also acknowledged that the tumor had metastasized to a pelvic lymph node on each side, which was more concerning, but all in all I felt relieved that the cancer hadn't spread to other organs outside the pelvis. And there was no spread to the bladder or rectum, which from my symptoms was the news I was expecting to hear. I left the doctor's office feeling a mix of fear, relief and confusion. On this day I also met the cancer care coordinator and the gynecological oncology psychologist, who would support me through my cancer journey. Their compassion, knowledge and humor gave me hope and confidence that I could begin this journey. They made appointments for a week later to meet with the radiation oncologist and the medical (chemotherapy) oncologist and assured me a plan was being put in place for my treatment.

Through the week, my biological sister was also Googling my diagnosis and came across posts on an online support bulletin board. It was by a lady called Angela from the US and talked about a Facebook group for women with my particular diagnosis. Within days I was a member of the group, and was among a group of around 60 other women and a couple of hundred supporters who had come together to provide information and support to other women faced with this cancer. It was so comforting to know I wasn't alone. And the group members were so positive and compassionate that I soon felt like I had all these new amazing friends who understood my journey and were there to support me through it. It also helped me to support the others, instead of solely focusing on the road ahead for me.

The next week I met with my treatment team. Firstly, the medical oncologist, whose obvious compassion and competence was comforting, but there was a negativity to the way in which she spoke which filled me with doom. She explained that the chemotherapy treatment was aggressive to meet the aggressive nature of the cancer, that the chemotherapy drugs would "weaken" the cancer cells, making them more susceptible to the radiation treatment, and the likely side effects were nausea, loss of hair, hearing loss and infertility. This was the biggest shock. The treatment would damage my ovaries, leaving me unable to have any more children. She countered my surprise by saying, "We are trying to save your life here." and, "We are throwing everything we have at this cancer." Due to the aggressive nature of the cancer they were expediting the treatment start date. I would begin combined chemotherapy and radiation in three and a half weeks time, which was ahead of the usual 5 weeks wait for treatment in our area.

Next I met with the radiation oncologist, whose competence and compassion was also clear. He had arranged for me to have a planning CT scan and information session early the next morning. He explained that I would have both external radiation and internal radiation (brachytherapy), which would occur simultaneously with the chemotherapy treatment. He confirmed that the radiotherapy treatment would damage my ovaries, leading to early menopause and damage the cells of my uterus so that it would no longer produce an endometrial lining and, of course, I would be infertile. He explained that the radiotherapy treatment was the best way to prevent the cancer from returning to my pelvis in the ovaries or uterus, which can often be a silent killer. I left the appointments feeling devastated about the loss of fertility, but relieved that there was finally a plan in place for me.

The next three and a half weeks dawdled. I just wanted to get that treatment started so I could feel in control, like I was doing something to beat this stupid cancer. It felt like every day I waited, that mass was growing bigger and bigger and spreading to other areas. Finally, the day I was to start chemo-radiation arrived and I went to the hospital. I was to stay on the oncology ward for the three days because of the highly toxic nature of the chemotherapy drugs. Over the next three months I received chemotherapy every 21 days. Cisplatin and Etoposide on the first day and Etoposide alone on the second and third days and then 18 days off, for my body to recover. I had two cycles of this followed by two cycles of Carboplatin and Etoposide on the same schedule. The Carboplatin was a less toxic drug and meant it could be injected at the chemotherapy day treatment centre. I coped pretty well with the chemo treatment, just experiencing some nausea and vomiting, loss of three-quarters of my head hair (my brother shaved the remaining, as it was falling out all over my clothes and bed linen and annoying me), and bathroom issues.

During the first month of my treatment, four women from the support group passed away. This shocked me and I came face to face with how incredibly life-threatening this cancer was. I wondered how much time I had left, how quickly my cancer would spread, how effective the treatment would be, and what would become of my two-year old daughter if the cancer took my life. I tried to take time away from the support group because the impact of lives lost so young was too much for me at the time. But I returned after several days because the positives of the support by the ladies, who I already called "sisters," far outweighed the fear that arose from acknowledging the reality of this disease. Over time, I read more of the ladies' stories and I was both saddened and inspired by their journeys and learned more about what I was up against in choosing to fight this cowardly beast.

Over the three months of treatment, I had twenty-five rounds of external radiation, where the radiation beam is directed at the pelvis and honed in on the tumor so as to produce as little damage to the surrounding tissue. At first it was disconcerting to have to lower my trousers and underwear to expose the area, while three or four strangers aligned the radiation machine and administered the ray. Sometimes I'd feel embarrassed, sometimes I'd cry, sometimes I'd try and focus on imagining the ray beams destroying those cancer cells. But the team was professional and would engage in conversation with me. Over the weeks it became just one of my daily tasks to perform. After five weeks of external radiation, I commenced three rounds of internal (brachytherapy) radiation. This involved three separate rods being surgically placed, under anesthetic, into the vaginal and uterine cavity, and high-dose radiation being emitted, proximal to the tumor and cervix. The surgical placement was painful, but the radiation itself was quick and painless. I burst into tears after the last brachytherapy because I was so relieved that this portion of the treatment was over. Even though I still had one round of chemotherapy remaining, my radiation oncologist reported that the MRI showed that the appearance of the cervix was just slightly abnormal at this stage. The tumor was almost gone!

During treatment, my diet changed dramatically, both through education regarding cancer and nutrition, and nausea, which prevented me from consuming previously enjoyed foods. I was eating mostly fruits and vegetables, a little lean meat, and had cut out all sugar and caffeine from my diet. I lost 13 kilograms during the course of treatment. After my treatment finished my mum, who was researching alternate cancer treatments, gave me a book called, Outsmart your Cancer by Tanya Harcourt Pierce, which became my bible in the aftermath of treatment. I ordered and began taking Protocel-50, a supplement on which there was a lot of positive information. I also added vitamin B17 to my diet. I took daily milk thistle tablets in an effort to rejuvenate my damaged liver cells, and twice daily Germanium tablet to enhance the cancer-killing capacity of the Protocel supplement. I had a lot of aches and pains and post-cancer fear told me it was the cancer returning, but a *scan at three months post-treatment confirmed that I was still clear of the cancer. Not only this, but examination by my oncologists showed that my pelvic area had a normal appearance and feel and showed no signs of radiation damage. The menopause symptoms of hot flashes, low mood and vaginal dryness started out moderate, but within three months became intolerable, so I began to take hormone replacement therapy in the form of pharmacist prepared bio-identical estrogen and progesterone. This has allowed me to live my life as though I am not yet menopausal, other then having no menstrual period, and the loss of fertility. The menopausal symptoms disappeared within weeks. There was much grief to process after treatment, but over time this has subsided. It has helped greatly to have the support of other ladies who have had similar experiences and to experience hope through the stories of survivors. While also knowing that the ladies who had fought so hard, but still lost their lives, had shared their stories and contributed to the knowledge that we, as a group, have about this deadly cancer. I feel ever so grateful to be here for my daughter, and want to continue to be a part of the "Sorority of Hope" sisterhood to support other ladies facing this cancer diagnosis. Together, I know we can contribute to finding the cause, and a cure for this dreaded disease, while raising awareness that a rare cancer would not otherwise receive. In a way, having a rare cancer was a blessing, as I often reflected during treatment. If I had a more common cervical cancer, I would never have been a part of such a group of beautiful, strong women who have supported me in this journey. It was that rareness that led me to seek support and find the group.*

The title of this story is not a reflection of any qualities of arrogance or complacence on my part, nor is it ignorance of the experiences of my small cell sisters who are suffering, or whose lives have tragically ended too soon, but it is a belief in the power of positive thinking and affirmation.

If you have read this story to this point, you probably would like to know if I beat this cancer, right? I'm now nine months post-treatment and, at this stage, am still cancer-free. It is still too soon to know whether I will survive. Apparently, doctors do not report a patient to be in remission from this cancer until the five-year mark is reached. It is just too unpredictable. My philosophy is that I will keep living my life, enjoying my life with my daughter and my family, making goals and plans for the future, until a scan or examination tells me I need to do differently. Either way, I know I'll be okay. The journey thus far has shown me just how loving and supportive my biological family truly is, and that I have wonderful friends who are there for me. I'm so thankful for all their hugs and caring words that helped me get through the treatment. I am also extremely grateful to the medical team that professionally and competently guided me throughout treatment. I also know that I have a wonderful group of women who share my hopes and fears, and that they will be by my side, emotionally–speaking, come what may. So I'll be okay - I've got my sisters!

Reference-*Harter-Pierce, T. (2009). Outsmart Your Cancer: Alternative Non-Toxic Treatments That Work. Thoughtworks Publishing: Stateline, Nevada.*

As this book got ready to go to print, our next sister lost her battle. She was a strong women and a true warrior of cancer.

We will continue to fight in her honor.

Becky Love's Story:

I was very much a latecomer to the sisterhood. In fact, it was 7 years after my diagnosis when I stumbled across a posting on a different cancer website from "Mum of 4 boys" in England, who, like me, also had Neuroendocrine Cancer of the Cervix.

Up until this point I hadn't looked into, researched, or spoken to anybody else who had the same diagnosis as myself and as I read through the posts and replies, I felt a connection to her. I saw her desperation, felt her pain and carried her fear from within, as only a person who has faced this can do. I read that she had been invited to join a Facebook page for other ladies with the same diagnosis and, as this was an old post and because of my own history, I felt that I needed to join and find out what had happened to this lady.

I found myself, all of a sudden, belonging to a group of ladies who were all going through or had been through what I had seven years previous, and they were all talking about it! I had never spoken to anyone. My oncologist had told me not to look online when it came to this cancer and I had listened to his advice. I have no real regrets over this, as at the time I was denied the knowledge that my survival rate after three years was 30%. I was blissfully unaware of how aggressive it was and shamefully ignorant of becoming metastatic. I well and truly buried my head in the sand and that is how I got myself through each day of the Hell that is cancer.

I was welcomed warmly into the group and as a long-term survivor, felt proud to be in a position of 'hope giver' to a beautiful group of ladies who had repeatedly been told by doctors that they wouldn't survive past two years. Doctors had been telling some of these ladies that there were no long-term survivors but I was living proof this was not the case. I began receiving private messages and it was a wonderful privilege to be able to give hope and some peace of mind to ladies who had been given no hope of a future. I don't suppose the reality of the diagnosis, even at this stage, had even fully sunk in. I was frustrated and angry and wanted these wonderful ladies to not listen to the doctors. I felt frustrated for them and wanted to shout, "I'm still here! I beat this, you can beat this!"

A vast majority of the ladies in the group were from America. I think at the time there were three in England, including myself, and a handful scattered in different countries around the world. Also, at this point in time, the sisterhood was for ladies with Small Cell Cervical Cancer and myself and 2 other ladies within the group had a diagnosis of Large Cell. It was one of these ladies, Rosie, who told me how very rare we were. One of only 5 ladies in the world, so she believed, and she had done her best to track us down. To receive all this information so long after diagnosis was very disturbing. I didn't so much sink into a depression but I found myself reliving everything I had been through. Even the realization that I had survived something so rare and aggressive hit me like a brick and the anxieties resumed. Of course I question myself as to whether I needed to put myself through this, but it was too late. I had met these ladies and was with then on their journeys and walking away wasn't an option. I had lived this for seven years and suddenly I wasn't alone.

Some of the ladies were open and honest, needing advice and solace for what they were going through. I sat and cried at their posts and responses, revealing intimate secrets of bleeding during sex, incontinence, vaginal scarring, etc. All these things I had lived through alone, too ashamed to share with anyone else. But not only that, having nobody else that had been through the same that could come anywhere close to understanding how I felt. It was a weight lifted from my shoulders and at last I could talk.

Several months passed before we started losing the first sisters since I had joined. It was sickening. Beautiful ladies, young and not so old, were losing their battle to this awful disease and nothing could stop it from happening. Children were losing their mothers, parents were losing their daughters and husbands their wives to a pointless death. As cancer sufferers we do suffer, believe me. It's not only the physical pain we have to endure, of which at times there is plenty. We watch those around us suffer, as relationships are broken just because of the strain of living cancer. Children lose us before we are even gone. Happy and carefree is no more, activities become a chore or even too painful to carry out. And we have the added burden of guilt to carry around that we did this to our loved ones and that once we are gone their lives will never be the same again. We can't be here to help them through their grief and they will suffer long after our deaths.

"Mum of 4 boys" had died not long before I joined the group, so I never did meet her.

I was 32 when I was given the news I had cancer. I sat in the doctor's office and nodded my head as a solitary tear rolled down my cheek. I looked at my sister and she looked at me and I just sat there listening to this voice, whilst in my head I was trying to process this information and think of the implications for myself and my children. The doctor was still talking and the word hysterectomy came out of his mouth and my world fell off its axis. I knew what a hysterectomy was and the implications but my brain refused to absorb the information and was searching for another meaning. I was repeating the word in my head thinking this isn't what it means, and that's when I broke.

The cancer didn't get me but losing my fertility felt like the end of world to me. I had 2 children and had separated from their father 3 years previously. I was desperate to marry and have a bigger family, it was my dream to have 4 kids from a young age and I never doubted it would happen. I saw fear reflected in the eyes of every person close to me and my own fear became out of control. I was a rabbit caught in the headlights and my body would shake uncontrollably, which made it just one more thing I didn't have control of. I didn't want this fear. I didn't want this cancer. It was somebody else's life because this isn't how my life was supposed to be.

I waited just one month for surgery and I cried the whole time. My relationship with my parents was strained and when, just 1 week after surgery, I was called in for 6 weeks daily radiotherapy and my mother told me to get hospital transport rather than take me, I knew I was on my own in this.

There was nothing that could prepare me for the pain and

suffering I went through over the following months. Every evening until the early hours were spent on the toilet, passing what I can only describe as acid laced with tiny shards of glass, over and over. My bottom was in tatters and the pain was unbearable. On top of this I had two children to care for. I couldn't wait the full, recommended 6 weeks of not driving because I had to take them to school and pick them up. Not lifting so much as a kettle was a joke because I had a house to clean and food to cook and every morning return back to the hospital for more radiotherapy. I am forever grateful for my Dad and the group of people who pulled together at the start to take me to these appointments and sit with me because these where the only times I didn't feel alone.

An irreversible connection with my mother was lost at this point. I have a daughter and there isn't a force in this world that would stop me being by her side every step of the way if she were ill. At home it was just my children and me and I took all that was thrown at me and refused to break, but I will never understand a mother who can walk away from that. Just simple things like cooking us meals and cleaning the house would have made my life so much easier. Nothing could take away my fear or pain but these were simple things and to have the help and support at home would have made a huge difference to our lives. Although I was ignorant to the full meaning of my diagnosis, cancer still to me meant death and the fear consumed me. I lay in bed at night shaking and really alone in the world. I had nobody to hold me or talk to or share this with and I don't think my brain/body/soul could take any more before it went into shut down. I had survived a surreal experience.

One night, as I lay consumed by fear and crying, a voice in my head told me that I was going to get through this and I can only compare it to the poem, "Footsteps", where there is only one set of footsteps in the sand and God told the burdened man "This is where I carried you". I woke the next morning feeling my burden lifted. I still had my fear and trauma. No one who has ever been diagnosed with cancer will escape that but I didn't doubt that I would be okay after that night. I just knew.

Seven years after diagnosis, to the month, a scan picked up a lump behind my bladder. Bad advice and an incompetent surgeon brought me back to the world of cancer. I feel I can say this with the information I have. No precaution should have been taken with my history. My bladder should have been completely removed with lump and clear margins. My surgeon went in and cut me up in strips, separating my bladder from the adhesions behind until he cut through the cancer, spreading it throughout my body. I waited just six months to be told I was terminal.

My name is Becky Love, and I am dying from Metastatic Sarcoma as a direct result from the radiotherapy I received, over eight years ago, to cure my Large Cell Neuroendocrine Cancer of the Cervix. But I am still a large cell survivor and nothing can take that away from me, I beat those odds.

We have many sisters from other parts of the world and we are grateful for all they do and love them through their journey. Being told "you will never meet another living soul with this diagnosis" only lent to the perseverance of many of these women in the group. Without this diagnosis we probably never would have met any of these women and now no matter where we go in this big, cold world, we know we are not alone.

Chapter 5

Our supporters, from the start, have been a huge factor in keeping this group going. They walk a different journey and see this diagnosis through eyes only they can. It is as important to these supporters to be a part of our group as it is for us to have them. These are the people that, in our darkest days, held our hands, prayed for us and stood by feeling helpless, yet never fled. Many of our supporters have lost their loved ones to this battle, yet they continue to love and support each of us who still fight. They continue to support funding for our project for research and they continue to help bring awareness to SCCC/LCCC.

Donna's Story:

Losing Rosie

By Donna Lindberg

Sept. 14, 2012

We didn't really lose Rosie. She has not been misplaced and we can't go looking for her and find her, as she was, alive and well, talking and smiling. We know where she is, in the University of Minnesota's anatomy lab. Rosie died early in the morning on December 27, 2011, one day before her 34th birthday, after an almost two-year battle with cancer. And not just any cancer. A rare, aggressive cancer. A cancer that has no cure.

I am the one who is lost without Rosie. She was my best

friend. We talked two or three times a day, every day. We were almost inseparable from the day she was born. And now, just 34 years later, my friend, my confidant, my precious baby is gone. It doesn't seem real somehow. Parents are not supposed to bury their children. It's like a part of me has been ripped away and that part is my heart.

Rosie wrote me a letter to open after she died. It took me about a month to get the courage to read it. I cried at all the beautiful things she said, but they also made me feel good. I was in awe of her ability to write this letter so soon before she died and to talk about what she wanted us to do after she was gone:

"Dear Mama,

I hate that you have to read this and go through this pain, but hopefully this letter can give you some comfort because it is wrapped in love. You've been the most loving, caring, tremendous, amazing, fantastic mother. I just really hope you never have to read this."

Rosie was born on December 28, 1977, in Minneapolis, Minnesota. She was a lively, healthy baby who was the center of my life from that day forward. When she was only three years old, her father and I were divorced. Rosie and I continued to live together, for 22 years, in the little two-bedroom bungalow in south Minneapolis where she was conceived.

Rosie's letter continued:

"I have nothing but good, warm memories of our life together in that house on 45th Avenue...of playing outside with neighbor kids while you did yard work; picnics on the

deck; being freaked out by storms (mostly you!!); walks on perfect summer nights; cuddling on the front porch; fun family birthday parties. I can only hope my own kids will be able to cherish memories like I had.

Oh, such a charmed life! Why didn't I know it was charmed at the time?"

Rosie grew to be a sunny, warm child and her name fit her perfectly. She made people feel special and she had many friends, many of whom were by her side at the end. She was also a real ham! She loved to perform, early on at ballet and piano, and later in many community and school plays. Rosie was a pretty easy child to raise, until she was 13 when she got into some trouble and almost got expelled from school. She turned herself around by her junior year of high school and eventually won a scholarship to Hamline University in St. Paul, where she studied theater and communications. Even during her difficult teenage years, we'd fight and make up, but we never stopped talking to each other. We shared everything.

Rosie went on in her letter:

"I know that after your divorce you were really struggling as a single mom. I totally understand now that I have my own kids. I praise you for being an amazing, wonderful, hardworking mom."

Rosie left home for the first time in 2001, to get an associate degree in zoo management at a school in Florida. In 2003, I moved from our little house in Minneapolis to West St. Paul to live with my dear friend, Del. Rosie and her boyfriend, Will, moved back to Minnesota in 2004, and Rosie got a job as interpretive guide on the monorail at the Minnesota Zoo.

I loved having her back home and our close bond was never again broken by distance or conflict...until now.

In the spring of 2007, Rosie told me she was pregnant. I was a little worried since she and Will were not married and neither of them had full time jobs. But I was also excited to become a grandma! On September 14, 2007, my grandson, Prince William Faulk, was born. Prince was a very special little guy, but his "special" status didn't last long. Isis Rose Faulk was born only 14 months later and she was very special too. I discovered that I had enough grandmotherly love for both of them. A good thing, since those two little motherless babies need a lot of my time and attention now.

Rosie was a good mom but having two babies so close together was hard on her, especially when she got sick. She wrote in her letter:

"Now that I have my own kids I have such a HUGE respect for you and everything you have done for me. I am so blessed and thankful you were there for me throughout my pregnancies and births. Now that they are here you have showered Prince and Isis with soooo much love."

My life was going along smoothly and I was pretty happy. Then everything changed in an instant. In March 2010, Rosie announced that she would be having a hysterectomy to remove a growth on her cervix...a cancerous growth that had grown to the size of a grape in only 11 months after a clean PAP smear.

Cancer. The Big C. I thought Rosie was perfect. How did she get cancer? There had never been much cancer in our families. Was it hereditary? Why hadn't I gotten it? Was it something I did? Did I feed her the wrong foods? Did I poison her with cleaning products and other chemicals?

Cancer was not a good thing to have, but surgeons removed all traces of cancer in Rosie and the 29 lymph nodes that were removed were also cancer free. We were sure she would recover and no trace of her cancer would remain. We were less sure when her doctor told us that her tumor was a very rare, aggressive form of cancer called Large Cell Neuroendocrine Carcinoma. He said there is very limited data on this cancer and only about 50 percent of people survive it. They knew of only about five other women worldwide who had the same cancer as Rosie and only about 40 with the small cell version of the disease. We were very scared and Rosie felt very alone.

We started to do some research on the disease online. We didn't find much and what we did find was not encouraging. Rosie wanted to know more about the other women who had this cancer. She wanted to talk to them, to meet them, to find out about their condition and prognosis, but her doctors could not give her their names.

She started a Facebook page in the summer of 2010, and through Facebook, finally connected with a couple of other women in different cities who had the small cell version of her cancer. These women were communicating with each other through a Facebook page called "Small Cell Carcinoma of the Cervix: Sisters United." Even though they didn't have the exact same cancer as she did, the prognosis for both cancers was similar and it was being treated in similar ways. She was now part of a club, the kind of club she wished she didn't have to belong to, but once she did, was the best thing for her. Suddenly she wasn't so alone.

She could talk to women who were going through similar treatments, suffering from similar side effects and scared like she was.

Rosie wrote on the "sisters" page in November of 2010:

"Rosie Fiercefighter Lindberg-Lakso

Hi Ladies,

I am so thankful to be invited to be a part of your group; you have literally been a lifesaver, true angel ladies!!!! After I was diagnosed on March 17 with Large Cell Neuroendocrine Carcinoma of the cervix, I couldn't find anyone else around who had this type of cancer or anyone who knows how to treat it.

God Bless you all and more power to you in your fight against your cancer!!!!!!!!!!"

A few months after Rosie joined the "sisters" page, two women with the same large cell version of Rosie's cancer joined the group and the title of the page was changed to "Small/large Cell Carcinoma of the Cervix: Sisters United." This helped Rosie bond even more closely with her "sisters."

Rosie was very lucky to have the best of care during her cancer treatment. She did not work full time at the Minnesota Zoo and, therefore, wasn't eligible for insurance coverage. As a low-income, single mother, she qualified for Minnesota Care, a state-run health insurance plan for people like her. Before starting her treatment, Minnesota Care reviewed her case and approved coverage of all her cancer-related care from that point on. They were good to their word on this and Rosie never paid more than a few dollars on co-pays, lab tests or hospital procedures. The

HMO that Rosie chose for her coverage was Park-Nicollet Methodist Hospital in St. Louis Park, Minnesota. Her cancer doctors, Dr. Peter Argenta, gynecology, and Dr. Michaela Tsai, oncology, worked at the Frauenshuh Cancer Center, connected with the hospital. These doctors had excellent credentials and together, they formed a team for Rosie's case that included consulting doctors from the M.D. Anderson Cancer Center in Houston, Texas, a clinic that had some limited experience with neuroendocrine carcinoma.

On May 24, Rosie started a six-week regimen of Cisplatin chemotherapy plus radiation. The main side effect from the chemo was fatigue that would knock her down for three to four days at a time. She barely had enough energy to go to work on weekends and she called in sick some days. A fund was set up on her Rosie "Fiercefighter" Facebook page so people could help her and Will with the financial hardships they were facing.

Rosie completed this first round of treatments on July 7, and got six weeks off in July and August. On August 3, 2010, she wrote her first entry on a Caring Bridge page she'd set up to keep friends and family updated on her condition:

"I've been enjoying my break from treatment very much. Playing with my kids, working, going to the cabin and to lots of parties. I'm having some hot flashes and mood swings, the hysterectomy caused me to go through menopause at age 32! Other than that I have really been feeling wonderful!!! I'm soooooo blessed."

On August 10, a PET/CT scan showed Rosie was cancer free, but she still had to return for four more rounds of double dose chemo, Cisplatin plus Etopocide, through mid-October. It was sort of the chemical equivalent of being hit by a truck. She got nauseated, lost her appetite and had a tough time taking care of her kids and working, but her bone marrow and blood counts remained high. Her spirits remained high too and she really believed she could beat her cancer.

Rosie finally lost her hair at the end of August and she was bald for her son, Prince's third birthday party on September 14. She showed off the cute, blonde wig she had gotten from the American Cancer Society and then posed bald for photos sitting next to her dad. They looked like twins!

In September 2010, I retired at age 63. I had always looked forward to retirement so I could have less stress in my life and travel more, but now I had a very different purpose for my free time. I can't imagine now what Rosie would have done if I hadn't been as available to take her to treatments, help with the kids and be there for her emotionally.

Oddly enough, I now cherish the many hours I was able to spend with Rosie while she got her chemo treatments at the cancer center. We'd chat endlessly, watch soap operas, work on our computers, drink gallons of coffee and eat the hospital's wonderful mushroom brie soup. Then, if Rosie was feeling well enough, we'd go to Caribou for, you guessed it, more coffee and maybe do a little shopping in the local stores. Again, it was a charmed time.

In mid-October, after Rosie finished her final round of Cisplatin and Etopocide, a CT scan showed that she was free of cancer. Rosie was elated. She took the kids trick or treating for Halloween and even she and Will dressed up in costumes. But the real monster was lurking, ready to strike.

In early November, Rosie began experiencing a pain in her right side that she thought was a strained muscle. She went to get a massage, but the pain didn't go away. Her oncologist moved her February PET scan to January 5. Rosie tried to get through the holidays with a smile, but I know this was weighing on her as it was on all of us.

On January 1, 2011, she wrote on her Caring Bridge page:

"Lord, I pray that you can give me and my family continued strength to accept the results of this scan and give me the strength to continue to fight and move on with my life."

I, too, wanted to believe, as she wanted to believe, that her scan would come out as clean as it had in October. But no such luck. The PET-CT scan had found a tumor in a rib on Rosie's right side and also an enlarged lymph node in her neck.

I was with Rosie on January 6, 2011, when she got the news. Her doctor told her she would need more treatments, but her cancer was incurable and they could only slow down the cancer's progression and maintain her quality of life. I wonder if Rosie ever understood or believed this. I know I didn't. She heard the words and cried. I heard them too and held her hand. A few minutes later, I ran to the bathroom and got sick. She had always worried more about me in all this than about herself and after the diagnosis I heard her pray, "Don't do this to my mom."

I was depressed for many days, but I knew I had to rally and help Rosie with her fight ahead. After the initial shock, Rosie too rallied and developed a fighting spirit and a determination to live life to the fullest and find some peace.

On January 11, 2011, she wrote on Caring Bridge:

"F*** YOU CANCER!!!!!!! YOU HAVE MESSED WITH THE WRONG WOMAN!!!!! MY BODY IS STRONG I CAN FEEL IT!!!!!!! I AM A SEXY TIGRESS!!!!!!!!!!! ROARRRRERRRRRRRRRR!!!!!!!!!!!!!"

The announcement of her diagnosis brought an overwhelming response from her friends and family and, of course, her cancer "sisters." A few days later, she again wrote on Caring Bridge and the "sisters" Facebook page:

"You just don't understand how overwhelming all of your support is to me. I feel wrapped up in a prayer blanket and I am all warm and cozy!!!! Peace is settling in."

In February, Rosie began radiation treatments for her rib tumor, followed by a new single-agent chemo, Taxol. The radiation reduced the pain in Rosie's ribs almost immediately, but she began to feel an enlarged lymph node in her chest. The hopes were that chemo would now shrink the lymph nodes. During these treatments, Rosie was a real "Fiercefighter" and went on with her life, worked at the zoo and took care of her kids. But it was then that I started thinking the unthinkable, about the possibility of losing my daughter.

The anniversary of Rosie's first cancer detection, March 17, came and went and miraculously, results from a scan showed that her lymph nodes were now normal size and the tumor on her rib was gone. There was a very small spot on her right upper lung so her oncologist continued her Taxol treatments until the end of May.

Rosie still did believe that one day she'd be free of cancer.

On her Caring Bridge page she posted this Bible verse:

"Exodus 23:25 Serve the Lord and healing will be yours, so you shall serve the Lord your God, and He will bless your bread and your water. And I will take sickness away from the midst of you."

This was another charmed period. Rosie and I went to New York City April 15-18 for the OMG (Oh My God!) young people's cancer summit. There, we had dinner with about 8 of her small cell "sisters" from all over the U.S. as well as Canada and Norway. Rosie said that this was the most important day of her life since she had been diagnosed. We attended only parts of the conference and then went sightseeing...to the top of the Empire State Building in the rain, ate lunch watching the skaters at Rockefeller Center, strolled in Central Park and took the subway to Wall Street and Greenwich Village. I have such wonderful memories of this last trip with Rosie. She was in good spirits and felt great. But the conference was sobering too, to be surrounded by over 300 people under the age of 40 with cancer. Meeting her cancer "sisters" and other cancer sufferers, survivors and friends at this conference gave Rosie and I strength as well as empathy and understanding of what others were going through.

Shortly after our return from New York we had a wonderful visit from a woman from the U.K., Beverley, who has the same large cell version of Rosie's cancer. Being able to meet someone who had the same cancer was very important to Rosie. Shortly after that, she also started communicating with Jen, another "sister" with her large cell cancer.

At the end of June, Rosie had another CT scan that showed

an increase in the size of the lymph node in her chest and more radiation therapy was scheduled. I think this was a real turning point emotionally for Rosie. She started to realize that she would never be cured of this cancer and she was having a hard time dealing with that.

She wrote on her Caring Bridge site:

"I don't expect to be "cured" from this cancer, but maybe maintain it for several years. God makes miracles happen, and they are plentiful!!!!!"

I could see Rosie's optimistic, fighting spirit waning and this broke my heart. She was getting very frustrated and depressed with living in limbo, not being able to move forward with her life or marry her now fiancé, Will. She was also getting desperate and looking for answers, cures, hope anywhere she could find it. She started seeing a therapist, Winnie, who introduced her to the Healing Codes that uses the body's immune system to naturally fight against disease. After one of her visits with Winnie, she came home looking happier and told me, "I am going to stop wasting time and start having fun with the beautiful life I have!!!"

But Rosie did not have time to live a fuller, more enjoyable life. In the fall of 2011, she developed a persistent, dry cough. CT scan results showed that the cancer had spread to her lungs and liver. The day she told me this, I was at the Minnesota State Fair. I tried to call her all day, but all I got was her voicemail, preceded by this Sting song:

"On and on the rain will fall like tears from a star, like tears from a star. On and on the rain will say how fragile we are how fragile we are."

When I finally did reach her, her tone of forced gaiety made it clear that her news wasn't good. She told me that she had gotten "the talk" from her doctor that she didn't want to hear, that she was getting to the end of possible treatments she could try.

In her September 9, 2011, Caring Bridge entry she said:

"WHATTTTTT, NOOOOOOOOOO I still have some fight left in me!!!! I am scared out of my mind and I am not ready for my babies to not have their mommy. My body is trying to give up, but my mind is not. Please give me your strength in prayer. I am not dead yet, and far from it. I am a Fiercefighter and I am going to do my best. Love you all sooooo much."

After getting "the talk," Rosie got a little frantic. She fought the toll the cancer was taking on her body by trying to do too much. One day, she vacuumed, cleaned the floors, took care of her kids, went on a walk and made chocolate covered strawberries. That night, she got very sick with a fever. It turned out that she had an infection and her doctor prescribed antibiotics. While she was recovering, I took her kids to the park where I met a woman, Julie, who said she was a healing nutritionist. Julie also said she worked for a doctor who had cured many advanced cancer patients with bio-feedback and other alternative methods. Rosie joined us at the park and met Julie and her husband, who held her and prayed for her. Rosie took this as a sign.

Rosie wrote on Caring Bridge:

"As they prayed for me the tears streamed down my face, the sun was setting beautifully in the west, the full moon was rising in the east, my children's voices were laughing and the wind started blowing hard!!!! There was my sign from God, that I had asked for, a renewal of peace, strength, health, hope, faith. Today was one of the most amazing days of my whole life. Thank you God for once again sending me your angels and your power to renew my fight and strength and direction."

Rosie went to see Julie's biofeedback doctor a few times, but she felt uncomfortable with him and thought he was kind of a quack. She did start making changes to her diet, drinking Julie's alkaline water, eliminating sugar, chemicals, dairy, red meat, and eating an organic, macrobiotic diet of mainly vegetables. I helped her shop for these foods and cooked her many meals.

She hadn't totally given up on traditional medicine though. She asked her doctor about getting a bone marrow transplant and was told that her body had to be free of all tumors before it could be done. Rosie agreed to continue with a new chemo, Navelbine. Her doctor also took a tissue biopsy to determine if a targeted treatment could be tried, but there was not a suitable match.

After Prince's fourth birthday in September, Rosie's cough and shortness of breath got worse. Her doctor prescribed an inhaler and Prednisone. The Navelbine, which wasn't working, was also stopped. At that appointment, Rosie signed an advanced directive that she didn't want aggressive resuscitative measures. Her doctor also discussed palliative care and hospice.

In October, a new PET scan showed that her cancer was spreading everywhere and her doctor told her that she had reached the end of her options. On her Caring Bridge page, Rosie said:

"I have come to the end of chemo and radiation. And I thought the tears and worry would start flowing everywhere, but no, almost a sense of relief. But not a relief to die, but a relief to let God take control completely. I feel so free with an amazing sense of peace. Love you all for your continued support and prayer."

Rosie began seeing a palliative care doctor for what she called her "next healing adventure!" In her last Caring Bridge entry on November 12 she was still upbeat:

"I am still here doing what God planned for me!!!!! Western medicine thinks I am dying and holistic and spiritual people think I am doing great!!! My therapist Winnie has helped bring peace and focus back into my heart, because some days can be soooo scary. I want to thank you all for the amazing prayer chain. It filled me with the light, life, and love of God and I could feel my cells soaking up his grace. I love you all so much and continue to feel your love, prayer, and protection."

Rosie did agree to try a new experimental chemo in pill form. The prescription cost her nothing, but the price listed on the package was $5,400. Unfortunately, these pills made Rosie very sick and she stopped after taking only three. She told her doctor then that she wasn't going to poison her body again, but she was still open to trying alternative remedies.

She did agree to see a Chinese doctor who was recommended by her stepmom, Sue. There she got an acupuncture treatment followed by a relaxing massage. She was also given herbs to take home, but the herbal tea made with them tasted terrible. She never went back for more treatments or more herbs.

On Thanksgiving, Rosie told me she was too weak to drive to our house for dinner. Del, his daughter Sarah and I packed up the organic turkey and side dishes I'd cooked and took dinner to Rosie. She told Sarah then that she couldn't imagine dying when she had so much spirit. "It's like I have all this life in me, but my body is just not cooperating."

I couldn't imagine her dying either and I was going to do everything in my power to stop that from happening. I made an appointment for her for early December with a specialist at the Penny George Institute for alternative medicine in Minneapolis. I spent five hours at the Park Nicollet Methodist Hospital medical records department getting copies of all Rosie's records for this doctor to review. But when the date of the Penny George appointment came around, she didn't want to go. I don't think she could find the energy to leave the house, even though part of her still believed a miracle would happen.

Since Rosie's diagnosis, I had bought 25 books about people who had beaten the odds and survived terrible cancers, looking for ideas, for treatments Rosie could try. I found an article online about alternative cancer remedies, including mushrooms from Taiwan that had been proven to shrink even advanced tumors. Rosie said she was interested in trying these so I bought her a bottle of 500 capsules for $700. She was supposed to take 20 capsules a day, but she only took five pills total out of that bottle.

I continued to cook macrobiotic meals for her that she didn't eat. She still drank alkaline water and the juices I made for her with wheat grass that was thought to have healing properties. But one day Rosie told me to stop trying to do so much. What she wanted for me was peace. And she just wanted me there for her spiritually. I was crushed. I think I really believed I could still save her life. I was still in denial.

Now I wish I had spent more of that time just sitting and listening to Rosie tell me her fears, her regrets, her belief in an afterlife, whatever was on her mind. But I was too afraid myself. It was her counselor, Winnie, who gave her advice on how to talk to her kids about her death. After that meeting, Rosie told me that she wasn't really afraid of dying, she had a strong faith, but she wasn't really at peace with it. She didn't want to leave her babies.

The last time Rosie left her house was to attend her daughter Isis' third birthday party on December 3, at a farm near our home. But she had trouble breathing and was barely able to get out of the car and into the door of the party room. But this was a good day, too, because all of her friends were there with their children and they had their picture taken together for the last time.

On December 9, Rosie went to the hospital emergency room because of pain in her chest. X-rays showed that she had fractured ribs from coughing. But she and Will had spent the whole night in the emergency room and Rosie came home exhausted. The next day, at the urging of her palliative doctor, Rosie began hospice care. I think she was relieved to be getting care at home.

On December 17, Rosie's friends held a fund-raising benefit for her at a downtown Minneapolis bar. Three bands donated their time to play that night. An auction was set up at the event and a silent auction was also ongoing on her Rosie "Fiercefighter" Facebook page. The funds raised helped Will and the kids get by for many months.

Rosie still kept looking for hope, for some kind of cure, for a miracle. A co-worker of hers knew a spiritual woman who she said had cured many people with the "laying on of hands." She was interested in trying just about anything and invited the women over. I was there, putting Isis and Prince to bed, and I could hear the two women quietly praying over Rosie while she sobbed. At that moment, I could actually feel my heart wrenching in my chest.

Despite her fears and determination to fight her cancer to the end, Rosie did start to get her business in order and prepare us for her passing. She said in her letter to me:

"When I am gone I will need you to help raise my children and take the role of being the mama in their lives. I know Daddy (William) will be their main caregiver, but he will need a lot of help."

Something changed after hospice care started and Rosie's condition deteriorated very quickly. Her breathing got worse and an oxygen tank was brought in. She was getting weaker and finding it hard to leave the house, even for radiation to reduce the size of the enlarged lymph node in her neck. She had a panic attack one day when I came to drive her to her appointment. "I'm so scared, I'm so scared, I'm so scared," she said and we held each other tightly. We cried together and I said, "What will I do without you?" But Rosie recovered quickly when Isis ran in crying, "Don't cry mama." Rosie comforted her saying, "It's okay baby. I'm okay." I was amazed at how she was able to put her fears aside and worry about her children. That was the last day she went for radiation treatments.

The turning point came on December 19, when the hospice doctor visited. Rosie had asked the nurse the week before if radiation might be able to shrink some of the tumors in her liver and lungs, since it had helped reduce the size of the lymph node in her neck. The doctor explained to Rosie that because her tumors had taken over so much of her organs, it would be hard to do radiation and avoid hitting healthy tissue. He then showed her the very graphic images of the cancer's progression from her last CAT scan. It took her a long time to respond, but she finally asked the doctor how long it would be before she died and he said, "No more than a couple of weeks." Then she asked him how she would die. He told her that when her liver stopped functioning, she would slowly lose consciousness.

The doctor's news was the last straw for Rosie. After the doctor left, she had a panic attack and told me she was terrified of losing a grasp on reality. She resisted taking her anxiety medications after that. She had a panic attack again that night and the hospice nurse had to give her a shot to calm her down. Will and I were extremely angry with the hospice doctor for what he had told her and taking away any hope she had left. Yet I also knew why he had done it. To help her let go. He knew she was holding onto life by a thread and it was time for her to die.

Five days before she died, Rosie asked Will to call everyone so she could say goodbye. Throughout the day, all her friends and relatives trickled in and out of her room to sit with her, hold her and talk to her. Food was brought in and everyone sat on the living room floor looking at Rosie and Will's photo albums. It was a very good day for Rosie and all of us, sort of a living wake.

The next day, the hospice nurse gave Rosie something to sleep since she had not slept for two days. She was afraid to go to sleep, she was sure she'd never wake up if she did. The lack of sleep, however, was adding to her anxiety. She slept for more than 13 hours that day, holding tight to the rosary our friend Luann had given her and a heart-shaped, pink stone given to her by her counselor.

On the Friday before Christmas, Rosie was having a harder time getting off the couch. Hospice came to insert a catheter and Rosie slept most of the time. On Saturday, Christmas Eve, we all gathered in the living room so that the kids could open their Christmas presents near her. She would respond when we talked to her, but rarely opened her eyes. Later, when Rosie was asleep, I saw Isis trying to put the Strawberry Shortcake necklace she had gotten for Christmas around her mom's neck. Rosie wasn't responding and I started to say, "Isis, don't…" then stopped myself. When Isis couldn't get the necklace over her mom's head, she draped it around her throat. Rosie didn't move the rest of the evening and the necklace didn't either.

On Sunday, Christmas day, the hospice nurse told us that Rosie would die in the next day or two. She also started giving her liquid meds that were injected with a syringe into her cheek. Pastor Carlson, from our church, visited Rosie that night, as did a faith healer that Will's family knew. Will said the next day, however, that Rosie had rallied to tell Prince that she loved him. She also talked on the phone to her best friend, Ellie, who lived in Portland. When Ellie cried and said she didn't want her to die, Rosie told her, "It's just my time, honey."

By Monday, we could no longer communicate with Rosie. But she never let go of her pink heart stone or her rosary. A few people visited, but didn't stay long. They all cried when they left.

I had a dream that night that Rosie and I were holding each other tight and crying as we floated above that couch where she lay dying. I wanted to do that, to hold her while she died, but she was not aware of anyone or anything those last few hours. She also was in obvious pain and sweating constantly. All I could do was hold her hand and wipe her forehead. I hope she knew I was there. I'd whisper in her ear that I loved her, but there was no flicker of recognition on her face.

That evening, Del and I took Isis home with us so Will could get a little break. It was easier for him with just Prince. At about 12:30 on Tuesday morning, December 27, Will called and as soon as I heard his voice, I knew Rosie was gone. I told him to call hospice and we'd be right over. I woke up poor little Isis and got her dressed. She chattered away obliviously as we drove the 25 minutes to their house. The hardest thing I have ever done was to walk into that living room and look at Rosie lying so still on that couch. I knelt down and kissed her and stroked her brow. She was still warm but her skin was very smooth and glassy. Her eyes were closed and she looked asleep, with no trace of pain or anxiety on her face. I remember thinking about this Dinah Washington song at that moment:

"This bitter Earth, that hides the glow of a rose. This bitter Earth, can it be so cold."

It had finally happened. My Rosie had died. But I didn't cry, I couldn't feel much. I just stayed next to her until the hospice nurse arrived to confirm that she had died. She called the University of Minnesota's anatomy lab. Rosie's last, selfless act of love was to bequest her body to research.

It took the U staff almost two hours to come so we had some quiet time with Rosie. After she was gone, Will came down with Isis. Prince had slept through the whole night and all the commotion. As soon as Isis saw the empty couch, she asked me, "Where did mama go?" I told her that mama had gone to be with God, that she was an angel now. Her response was "Oh. Grandma, can you play with me?" So I played with her for a while and then we went home. There was nothing else to do and Will and the kids needed sleep. When I got home I didn't go to bed. I had tea and stared out at the approaching dawn and thought, "This is the first day of the rest of my life without Rosie."

This was the last entry on Rosie's caring Bridge site, written by Rosie's dad on Saturday, December 31, 2011:

"Rosie's Memorial Celebration

Rosalyn Julia Bessie Lindberg-Lakso

Dec. 28, 1977-Dec. 27, 2011

Our dear Rosie lost her fight with cancer one day before her 34th birthday. Rosie's last wish was to have a celebration filled with balloons and roses where people can remember the happy times of her life. A memorial service with a reception to follow has been planned for January 4 at 11 a.m. at Christ Church Lutheran in south Minneapolis. Memorials accepted online at Rosie's Fund, the small/large cell cervical cancer M. D. Anderson project or the University of Minnesota Medical Foundation or Anatomy Bequest Program."

I spent the next few days in a daze. I didn't have much time to grieve. I had many things to do. And I don't think it had really sunk in yet that Rosie had actually died. It was still unreal somehow. I also think I felt a sense of relief. This made me sort of sad and also guilty, but I think I was glad that Rosie had finally been relieved of her physical and emotional suffering.

Rosie's memorial service was very nice and there was a large turnout. After the service, 33 balloons were handed out to the family to release…the number of years Rosie had been on earth. They were turquoise and white, the cervical cancer ribbon colors, and we watched them float up to space until we couldn't see them anymore. For the celebration that followed, we decorated with animal print balloons and ribbons. There were bouquets of roses and other brightly colored flowers in vases with feathers and beads and sparklers. Many people got up and shared memories of Rosie and a 300-slide show of her life was shown throughout. My friend Del's daughter, Sarah, read a memorial I had written for Rosie, since I knew I couldn't have read it myself. Elijah, a friend of Rosie and Will's, read the poem "Life is No Crystal Stair" by Langston Hughes. At the end, we played a recording of the song "Time to Say Goodbye," sung by Andrea Bocelli and Sarah Brightman:

"When you're far away, I dream of the horizon and words fail me. There is no light where there is no sun and there is no sun if you're not with me. Time to say goodbye.

Now I shall sail with you to places I've never seen upon ships across the seas, seas that exist no more. I know that you're with me. It's time to say goodbye."

Then it was over and the long, painful process of grief began.

I don't remember much of those first few weeks after Rosie died. I think I was in a dream, no nightmare, state. I just went through the motions. Now that eight months have passed, some of the bad memories of her last days are fading, but the grief, though less powerful, is still my constant companion. I think of Rosie as soon as I wake up in the morning until the moment I go to sleep at night. When friends ask how I'm doing, I tell them I still have this dull, gray feeling about life, like I'm in one of Stephen King's novels. Even though I go about my life as before, no matter where I go or what I do, there is always that "Dark Tower" in the distance. I've lost interest in so many things like traveling, activities or entertainment. My life revolves around little Isis and Prince now. They are my main reason for living.

I am still angry at the cancer that ravaged Rosie's body and the things in the environment that most likely contributed to her cancer; pollution, ozone depletion, chemicals, plastics, processed foods, genetically modified crops, hormones, pesticides and herbicides. I don't want my grandchildren to grow up and get sick from the foods they eat, the air they breathe or the things they touch. In the future, I want to donate any time or energy I have left to improving the environment.

I am still incredibly sad about the loss of dreams...of Rosie's dreams...of not seeing her children grow and change from year to year...of the many places she will not see...the wonderful career she could have had...the home she wanted. And my dreams...of not being able to go on trips with her...of the times we could still enjoy together...of not having her beside me when I die. So many dreams, gone with the wind.

Even at the end, when Rosie saw her dreams slipping away, she worried more about us than herself. In her letter to me she told us what to do with our grief. It is hard for me to imagine the strength it took for her to write this:

"You, William and the kids may need a great deal of emotional support right now. Please make sure the kids are showered with love and Mom, please make sure you leave time for you and accept the loving help and support that you need."

I know Rosie would want our lives to go on, so I try to get through each day and take care of myself, for my grandchildren. I know the grief, anger and regrets will one day begin to fade. In the meantime, I am learning something from them too...about life...about death...and about myself. I realize now, as I've said many times, that we all are living charmed lives. Rosie's illness and death, although tragic and too soon, is what we will all go through. We are put on earth for only a short while and we never know when it is our turn to say goodbye. I may experience many more tragedies and deaths before my own and they will change my life too. Now I feel that my life has more purpose, to love my family and friends more, to enjoy the beauty around me more, to love my life more. The author Isabel Allende, who lost her 28-year-old daughter Paula in 1992, has said that she is now a happy woman because her daughter's death taught her how precious life is. This is also my gift from Rosie, her life charmed me, and I know that, in time, her memory will allow me to be happy once again.

I have to acknowledge that I'm not the only person mourning Rosie. Will has his good and bad days, but he's doing his best to be both mother and father to Isis and Prince. They love him and seem to be happy, normal kids and this has become the "new normal" for them. Rosie's dad, Wayne, and stepmom, Sue, are always there for Will and the kids. Together, we co-grandparent our mutual grandchildren.

Rosie's friends miss her too. The day after she died, December 28, 2011, would have been her 34th birthday. Her friends invited me to a birthday party and we cried together as we lit the candles on a cake that said, "Happy Birthday, Rosie." Since then, I am always invited, along with Isis and Prince, to their get-togethers and children's birthday parties. On Valentine's Day, her best friend Adriana and I got tattoos in Rosie's memory. Mine is of a rose entwined around a heart that sits right over my own heart. Adriana's is of a large heart with wings just below her neck. We will take these symbols of our love for Rosie to our graves.

After Rosie died, I started to communicate with her cancer "sisters" on Facebook. I had met many of them when Rosie and I had gone to the OMG Cancer Summit in New York in 2011. I also met many new sisters online. Communicating with them was comforting to me and I also felt a need to provide them with the comfort and support I could no longer give Rosie. The sisters encouraged me to attend the 2012 OMG Summit in Las Vegas. So, at the end of March, I flew to Vegas and spent four wonderful days with some of the bravest, liveliest, awe-inspiring women I have ever known! When I arrived for dinner the first night, I was showered with hugs and kisses. During the time I spent with these women, I became inspired by those who were remaining cancer free, and sobered by the many who were struggling with the disease. On that trip, I was unofficially dubbed, "Mama Donna" and I am very proud of that title. I feel like all their mamas now and I want to wrap them all in my arms every day.

Since that trip to Vegas, I have continued to communicate with the "sisters" on Facebook and I have followed their postings about their cancer journeys, struggles and victories. Five of the sisters have died since Vegas and this took its toll on me. I told the sisters that I would not be going on the page as often as I did before; it kept bringing back painful memories of Rosie's last days. But I can't stay away totally. I have too much of a connection to them, too much love for them.

On Mother's Day, Isis and Prince and I planted gardens for their mom at their house and my house. We filled them with roses and colorful annuals. There is a little plaque in their garden that says, "Mom's Garden" and one at our house that reads: "The truest love is between mother and daughter." Rosie's cancer sister, Melanie, her sisters, Vicki and Toni, and their mom, Judy, visited us in July. They brought some lovely ornaments for Rosie's garden. We had a picnic on our porch and reminisced. Then we all had our picture taken around Rosie's newly embellished garden, a picture that I posted on the "sisters" page and on the "Remembering Rosie" Facebook page.

Little Isis and Prince are already saying that they are starting to forget their mom. This makes me sad and afraid. I'm starting to forget her, too, and I worry that it's too soon not to see her face and hear her voice. I am trying to create rituals for them like looking through photo albums. When they look at them, Isis says she misses her mom and Prince kisses her photos, but they are really too young to be sad. I use the albums to help me talk about things Rosie did or said. I also sing songs that Rosie used to sing to them like "Rockin' Robin," "Three Little Fishies" and "Ugly Duckling."

Rosie asked me in her letter not to let her children forget her:

"Please help them to never forget who I am."

No, Rosie, I will never let Isis and Prince or anyone else forget the wonderful, special person you were. I will tell them about your love for people, your warm personality and your love of life. I'll also tell them how much you loved being a mom and how much you loved them. And I'll also tell them about the wonderful times we had together and how much I loved you.

Oh how I miss you, Rosie, and I will say it with every breath I take until I can't take any more. You were my daughter, sister and best friend all rolled into one. You may have been only one person in a world full of billions, but you were the world to me. I so hope that I can see you again, that we can be together and hold each other.

Rosie's letter to me ended this way:

"Love you Mama so much. This is not goodbye."

This is the song I often sing to you now, Rosie:

I'll be seeing you in all the old familiar places that this heart of mine embraces all day through. In that small cafe; the park across the way; the children's carousel; the chestnut trees; the wishin' well. I'll be seeing you in every lovely summer's day; in everything that's light and gay. I'll *always think of you that way. I'll find you in the morning sun and when the night is new. I'll be looking at the moon, but I'll be seeing you.*

Rhonda Dixson-Perry's Story:

In August 2010, my beautiful, young niece, Candeese Dixon, and her dad, Vincent, received the horrible news that she had Small Cell Cervical Cancer. I was at work that afternoon when my mom called to let me know. After hearing the news, I left the office got into my car and mindlessly drove through the streets of Nashville, not knowing or caring where I was. I could not believe what I'd heard; my beautiful sweet, funny and sexy niece had cancer. We all knew Candeese was having issues with long menstrual bleeding and at the very worst we expected a diagnosis of endometriosis or fibroids. Never, in a million years, did we think cancer. But cancer it was. And not just cancer, but a rare cancer that we knew nothing about.

I wanted to find out everything I could about this disease and put her in contact with others who also had the disease. I scoured the Internet day and night and came across a couple of names. I found a story by Colleen Martlett and prayed that I could get in touch with her. I searched her name on Zabasearch to see if there was a recent contact for her, but there were many out there. I called a couple of them but got no answer and did not leave a message.

So I continued to search for other survivors and, thankfully, I ran across Angela Van Treuren. I emailed her and she immediately responded warmly to me. I immediately felt like I'd found a new friend. Angela told me about the

SCCC/LCCC Sisters Group on Facebook and Candeese finally joined.

This group was a Godsend, as Candeese was able to connect to people who, like herself, were battling this beast of a cancer. She immediately fell in love with Angela and she also forged a deep friendship with Pearlie, the only other African-American that was part of the group at the time Candeese joined. Candeese also drew strength from the other ladies of this group and, although she did not post every day, she read each and every one of the sisters' stories and postings. Candeese was grateful to meet Melanie Cummings, who I think of as the "Great Uniter." Melanie, a survivor of SCCC, seems to have made it a personal mission to meet as many sisters and supporters as possible.

In November 2011, Candeese learned that one of the sisters, Alyson Strong, lost her battle to this disease and I was concerned about her finding this out. But when she heard the news she said to me, "Auntie, this only makes me stronger."

Well she did get stronger. Not physically but spiritually, and her courage was a pillar of strength to all of us. Candeese never once asked why was this happening to her, but she did not want anyone else to go through this.

This is what my niece posted on Facebook:

"In August of 2010, I was diagnosed with a rare form of cancer called, Small Cell Cervical Cancer or Small Cell Carcinoma of the Cervix (SCCC).

SCCC: Does not come from HPV, so cannot be detected in a pap smear test

Affects 0.6% of females out of 100,000-any age, any race

Extremely aggressive & likes to metastasize to other organs in the body

Has a poor prognosis rate

I began treatment right away which included chemotherapy & radiation and in March of 2011, I was considered to be disease-free or in remission. Still, my oncologist wanted me to have scans every 3 months to keep a close eye on me. In June, I went in for my first scan & was told the sneaky cancer had returned & spread to my liver, lungs, lymph nodes & blood! My oncologist was afraid that this cancer was resistant to chemo, seeing she had given me the strongest therapy out there. So, not giving up, I began treatment again, using 3 different chemo drugs & added GOD to my treatment plan this round. As of now, I am currently in treatment & although the doctors are not certain if anything will work, I believe I am already healed. I am walking by faith and not by sight.

I was on FB a while back, deleted my account because I had no real use for it. This time I do. I want to use FB to keep my family & friends updated & connect with my fellow SCCC sisters all over the world! There's not many of us. I want to share my journey so that my testimony will be one for you. I know the doctors consider me to be "unhealthy" but spiritually & mentally I feel good. Don't get me wrong, I have my moments, I am human but now I rely on GOD and his word, which is more comforting than anything else. So, CANCER I BIND YOU IN THE NAME OF JESUS AND LOSE MYSELF!!! AMEN!"

On December 23, 2011, my niece was called to Heaven.

Every day I miss her, every day I shed a tear for her, but every day I have hope that a cure will be found, not only for small/large cell cervical cancers, but all cancers.

Many sisters and supporters have established fundraisers to help raise money for research; I have a Crowdrise page, in honor of my niece, to help support this effort. Candeese's dad wrote the following post on our fundraising page

"My daughter, Candeese N Dixon, recently lost her battle against Small Cell Cervical Cancer. During her journey she expressed that her fight was not just for her but for other SCCC patients, to instill hope in those who otherwise had little or no hope at all. The purpose of my donation is to help continue her fight against SCCC. Thank You, Candeese, for showing me how to fight,,,,,,,,,,,,,and to Love."

I am thankful to be a supporter of the SCCC/LCCC group. I rejoice for all victories both big and small. I am known as "Auntie Rhonda," which I embrace with love. Because I do love each and every one of these ladies and I know that there is a victory coming for us. We must never give up hope and, as they say, we all have to "Fight Like a Girl". I too am surviving this disease, although I have never received a cancer diagnosis of any kind. But survival comes in many forms and, as supporters, we have to survive every bit of bad news and rejoice in the good news and realize that hope exists as long as we can tell the story.

Toni Petoskey's Story:

It was May 2007. I got a phone call from my youngest sister. Mel has cancer. Cervical cancer. Small Cell cervical cancer. I cried and cried. I was beside myself. We had lost our Dad to small cell lung cancer in 2004. I knew small cell cancer was going to be a fight. I then had to call our oldest sister and tell her. More crying. I was trying to figure out what to do next. After many phone calls with my mom and my sisters, I decided I would fly to Mel in Michigan and help her through her treatments. As I was packing, just throwing things into my suitcase, I was crying. I was mad, I was hurt, I was angry. Why was this happening to our family again? I then Googled Small Cell Cervical Cancer. What I read was another blow to my brain. SCCC represents 3% of all cervical cancers; it is an aggressive tumor that spreads very quickly. They are often diagnosed in an advanced stage and their prognosis is poor. There are no clinical trials, due to their rarity. They treat SCCC like Small Cell lung cancer. I knew the outcome of this, as our dad battled it for 22 months. If she made it through treatment the chance of recurrence or metastases to the lung, liver and brain was high. Only 20% make it to 5 years. Right then and there I decided I would be right by Mel's side, holding her hand through this journey. Good or bad I would be there for her.

I got on the plane, flying from Atlanta, Georgia to Flint, Michigan. So much was going through my head. Mel didn't know I was coming. I was going there to surprise her. I knew she would be so happy I came. She works late hours at a hospital. I sat at my mom's kitchen table waiting for her to get home. I didn't know what I would say to her. I played it in my head a hundred times. She would hug me, we would cry, I would say I'm sorry and things would be ok. When she got home she walked right past me. She didn't see me sitting there. She walked right past me downstairs and spoke to my mom. She said, "I'm home. I'm tired and going to bed." On the way up the stairs she saw me sitting at the kitchen table. She said, "What the hell are you doing here?" I said, "I came to see you." She said, "I'm going to bed." That was it. I sat at the table for hours. Trying to wrap my head around what she must be going through. Ok, I won't ask her anything about the cancer. I will just be by her side to help her any way I can.

I stayed for two weeks to help her through her treatments. We spent that time together but didn't talk. I helped her with her meals and gave her medicine. I brought her water and snacks. I sat in her chair, next to her bed, in the dark, while she rested in her bed. Day after day, most of the time we sat in the dark and said nothing to each other. I thought she was so strong. She wouldn't let my mom, or me, drive her to treatments or to her doctor appointments. She drove. She also made the decision to still go to work. Strong, brave, whatever you want to call it, she was doing much better than I would have done. I left Michigan to go home for a few weeks and then flew back to help her for two more weeks. She was happy to see me the second time around. We talked, we laughed and we cried. One night while she was resting in her bed and I in her chair, in the dark not saying anything to each other for hours, she said, "If I make it through treatment would you go to Florida with me for a vacation?" I, of course, said, "Yes!"

I met her in Fort Lauderdale with our niece, Amanda. We had such a good time. As we sat out in the sun drinking fruity drinks I said to Mel, "Wouldn't it be great if we could do this every month?" She said, "I don't know about every month, but let's try the next 4 months." The next month I planned a trip to Disneyworld. Our Niece, Amanda, and our *older sister, Vicki, and our brother-in-law, Bob, came too. We had a wonderful time. We traveled each month for the next 4 months and decided to go to Key West for Christmas. We called it "Cancel Christmas and Go To Key West." No gift giving, just spending time with family. 2011 was our fifth year canceling Christmas and going to Key West. We have made so many wonderful memories. Mel and I traveled each month, for 15 months, after she finished treatment.*

On one of our many trips to Fort Lauderdale, Mel told me about a woman she had met online on Cancer Compass. She had the same cancer as Mel, and they shared the same birthday. I was so happy that Mel found someone she could relate to. Someone going through the same thing she was. Her name was Colleen and she lived in California. Colleen gave Mel hope and courage and Mel gave her the same. They had a bond. The two of them started a webpage called, "Cancer Comrades." It was a site for women with SCCC to connect and not feel alone. I was so proud of those two girls, e-mailing woman with the same disease as they had, knowing what the outcome could be. They met Angela online and they decided to make a Facebook page. In 2011, Angela found out about a cancer conference in New York. The girls talked about going and meeting. I think it would be the first time any SCCC/LCCC sisters would meet. Mel wasn't sure she wanted to go. She asked me to go with her. I said I would go. She still wasn't sure she should go. I told her she would regret not going to the first SCCC/LCCC meeting of the sisters. I would be there by her side and she would be ok. I knew meeting these sisters would be hard because it would be real and some might not make it. But I thought we should go.

We met for dinner the night before the conference. Nine women with SCCC/LCCC and their Sister Supporters in one room. I can't even tell you the joy in everyone's eyes. I just keep thinking in my mind, watching these sisters, this is their first meeting.

In New York, I met a girl from Minnesota. Come to find out she lived 10 minutes from my oldest sister. Her name was Rosie. She had LCCC. I also met a young girl named Ally, who lived in New York. She was 24 years old and new to the Facebook group. Then there was Becky from Virginia, Mona from Norway and Debbie from Canada. I was so glad we had made the trip. I knew it was going to be life changing. There was talk about meeting the next year at the conference and bringing more sisters together.

In 2012, 19 SCCC/LCCC sisters and Dr. F, who will be heading the research project at MD Anderson, and at least that many supporters met in Las Vegas. There were women from all over the world. It was the first meeting for most of them. I was lucky enough to be able to go and be a part of this wonderful weekend. This is where Mel and Colleen got to meet in person after first meeting online a few years before.

I have stayed in contact with many women I've met and made new sister friends and sister supporter friends on the Facebook page from all over the world. We have lost many since this group began. I know they are all angels, looking down on this wonderful sisterhood, sending love, support and guidance. I'm proud to say I'm a Small cell/ Large cell sister supporter.

By, Toni Petoskey

Cydney Marlett's Story:

I am not a supporter in the group, but I am a supporter of my mom. I was only in 8th grade when she was diagnosed with SCCC, so that is the main reason I am not in the group. I am now 20 and in college and I can share my experience, being the child of a woman I thought could conquer the world.

My name is Cydney Marlett and my mom is Colleen Marlett. When she first told my brother and me that she had SCCC, all I knew is she had cancer. All I knew about cancer was that my grandmother and biological grandmother had died from it. I was scared. Mom had never lied to us about anything. As far as moms go, judging from other families, my mom had always been very upfront and I could always talk to her about everything. So, when my brother interrupted her telling us about the cancer and said all he wanted to know was if she was going to die, I waited for her response and watched her carefully. I thought I would know for sure if she lied. She said she was not going to die, not at that moment, and did not intend to die from this cancer. I believed her. But deep down inside me, I was scared and worried.

I remember when her hair started falling out. I think that scared her and I wanted to comfort her. Her mom, my grandmother, had died a few years before from ovarian cancer and had left behind her braids from when she was a little girl and had cut them off at school. My mom was usually a blond but that last year, before she got sick, had gone to a dark red color, which was a lot like the color of my grandma's hair when she was little. Mom decided to shave her head when her hair started falling out. So we went outside by the pool, I weaved her long, curly hair into braids and made the cut. I think she still has those braids saved in the same bag as my grandmother's braids. I don't know why it was important for her to have my grandmother's braids after she died, or why she wanted her hair braided in the same way before losing it all. But I know she keeps them in a drawer in her room. This, for some reason, is the most vivid memory I have of that time and will always be with me.

Looking back, I also realize that while life was going on as usual for all of us, it wasn't for Mom. I am amazed now, thinking about all the treatments and surgeries she went through all on her own, because that is who she is. She didn't want it to touch us. Even though terrible things were happening anyway, she kept the worst from us. But I saw. I saw her run out her sliding doors in the morning and throw up. I saw her, pale and tired, getting up and driving us to school before she went to chemo. It made me mad. At who or what, I am still not sure. For the next 3 years she struggled through treatments and surgeries, PET scans and doctor's appointments. Then the cancer came back and we started all over. We had money troubles that my parents tried to keep from us, but as I got older, I could see for myself. The mom that was indestructible in my eyes was now in her bed and definitely did not look like the mom I had always known. She was there, but she had her own issues to deal with, so why bother her with mine? I think she thought everything was fine with me, as we had always been so close. Part of me just didn't want to bother her and another part of me was just being a teenager. Needless to say, our family suffered in many ways through this diagnosis and mom was left picking up the pieces after she became cancer-free the second time.

It has been a long road back to what was once normal for us as a family. I have changed because of the cancer and the choices I've made in trying to deal with my feelings. But things are better than they have ever been. What I thought might kill my mom has actually made her even stronger than before. There was a time when I thought she would beat the cancer but never be the same mom again. I was wrong. She is the same and more. We talk all the time about everything, as we once did, and she shares with me all the stories of her SCCC/LCCC sisters. Sometimes I wonder how she can continue to do what she does on a daily basis. But she says to me, "It is what I am supposed to do." I have heard her and Mel on the phone, talking for hours about the next thing they will do, always trying to spread awareness and raise money. I am always surprised when I hear them say they feel as if this is a "calling." I thought that only happened with priests and nuns. I have cried with her about every loss of a sister and watched her face as she tried to pull herself together enough to keep going on, and she always does. My mom is indestructible and she will conquer the world. But first I think she will conquer this disease, or at least give hope and inspiration to those who come to the group with this diagnosis. I love you Mom. Thanks for being such a great role model.

Melanie was reading a rough draft of this book and had left the manuscript sitting out in her room. Her mom had picked it up and read it, but didn't want Mel to know she had been reading it right away. She left a little note inside the book for

Mel, which said:

"I knew I had to do everything I could for you daily and God would take care of the rest. He is all-powerful. He is God.

I am so proud of your strength and determination and your commitment to this SCCC cause. I pray God puts his blessing on the book endeavors, that it may reach and help and comfort other cervical cancer patients and their families.

Remember, God is always with you! Love, Mom"

To our supporters: we are less than whole without you. Every day we thank God for you and all that you have done to love us through this diagnosis. Thank you for walking this path with us.

Chapter 6

These next stories are truly inspirational. Some of these women go back 4 or 5 years and some are newly diagnosed, but the voices behind these stories seem to be the same. There is no other place for us to go where someone can understand the diagnosis and the obstacles we face. So we share with you more stories of women battling today, as well as women who have won this battle and stand alongside those facing their first steps.

Here is Nicole's Story:

I'm Nicole, the anal sister. Seriously, I did not have this cancer in my cervix, like the others in the group. The cancer started in my rectum. And what a real pain in the ass it has been!

Around mid to late 2010, I started losing weight without trying. I have some Polish in me and have always had a butt. Not as big as Kim Kardashian's or anything, but not ever flat, that's for sure. I was especially losing my butt and muscle mass from my legs. I thought it was from stress, as I was going through a lot at the time. Then my energy started diminishing. In January 2011, it felt like I had a hemorrhoid, but I was not linking all of my symptoms together. The suspected hemorrhoid was up a few inches in my rectum. I tried self-treating for a few months, but the pain was getting worse and the treatments were not helping. By June it was getting pretty bad and I remember having an anxiety attack and not being sure why. Now, when I look back, I think it was because I knew something was seriously wrong and was too scared to admit it to myself.

I actually heard a voice (God, I believe) say to me while I was in the shower, "You have cancer." I tried to block it out and tell myself I was just being paranoid, but this wasn't the first time I'd heard that voice. It scared me into pushing harder to find out what was wrong with me, and that saved my life.

I went to my doctor, who told me he thought I had a fissure or cut in my rectum and gave me some cream to try. It didn't work so he tried antibiotics. Those didn't work either. In the meantime, the pain was getting worse. With every bowel movement I had so much pain I thought I would pass out. There was a ridge in my movements and it seemed obvious that a lump was causing that. It started hurting with every step I took and then I couldn't sit down without feeling pain. That's when I heard the voice while I was in the shower. "You have cancer." But I denied it and told myself I was just freaking out because of the weight loss and the hemorrhoid. But it made me push harder for an answer since that voice had been right in the past.

After several visits with no results, I finally told my doctor, "Something is seriously wrong with me! I'm not a hypochondriac!" That's when he scheduled me to see a surgeon. I felt desperate to get this thing out of me, but the surgeon just gave me some more cream to try. I kept insisting it was a lump, but he kept saying it was a fissure or an ulcer. On the next visit to the surgeon, I begged him to just take it out.

He said, "It's not cancer." I asked, "How do you know?" He

replied, "Because cancer there doesn't hurt." I actually felt a little relieved that he seemed so sure it wasn't cancer. I don't think he was imagining this rare, aggressive cancer that only strikes about 1 in 100,000 people. And, by the way, I've since spoken to a lady who had colon cancer and it certainly hurt her! They didn't want to do a colonoscopy on her because they said she was too young, even though she had a family history of colon cancer.

Anyway, the surgeon said he was going on holiday and I begged him to take it out before he left, telling him I couldn't stand it anymore. He told me I could go to the US and pay $15,000 and have it out tomorrow, but things didn't work that way here in Canada. I couldn't believe he was talking to me like that when here I was, almost in tears, asking him to just get it out. He finally took it out about 10 days later and told me it was an ulcer. I started feeling better within a few days.

"You have got to be kidding me! Please God, NO!"

After months of being told it was a fissure or an internal hemorrhoid or an ulcer, I got the dreaded call to come into my doctor's office. I had just been in the day before and was told the lump they took out of my rectum was an ulcer. Now my doctor was telling me it was cancer, and I had to see an oncologist right away!

My doctor told me, "Don't worry, it is a slow-growing kind." When I saw the oncologist a few days later, she said, "No, it's not slow-growing. The type you have is called Small Cell Neuroendocrine Carcinoma and it is very aggressive and fast-moving." She said it was so rare that she had only treated two patients with it during her entire career. She told me that there was no treatment protocol for this type of cancer so she was going to treat me as if it were small cell lung cancer. They scanned everything from my head to my bones and didn't see signs of cancer anywhere else. Thank God. They were not fooling around with this one.

The oncologist didn't tell me that this type of cancer is known to recur, but I found that out later. The lump had been taken out, but if even one undetectable cell had gotten loose, it could travel and spread anywhere. All of this information was quite shocking, as I had been feeling great since the lump was removed. The radiation oncologist assigned to my case consulted with several other radiation oncologists and they felt that, if I could handle it, they should do radiation at the same time as chemo to give me the best chance of a full cure.

"Are you kidding me? Oh my gosh, is this really happening?"

It was pretty shocking and scary. Of course, being the type that has to know everything, I Googled my diagnosis right away. I was even more scared after finding there was not much information out there and what I did find, didn't give me much hope. The anxiety was at an all-time high and I was having a hard time getting to sleep. Nighttime definitely seems to be when the Cancer Boogey Man comes out to play with your mind.

Chemotherapy started that Monday, on my husband's milestone 50th birthday. Happy birthday, Bruce. He was at my side for my first chemo session. In the past three weeks we had lost our best friend, Albert, to liver disease, made plans to attend his funeral, found out I had cancer and prepared to start chemo. And we were supposed to be ringing in Bruce's 50th?

We were numb and I was scared shitless. Between losing his best buddy and all that had been going on with me, Bruce was in a bad funk. He was so worried about losing me. I told him, "Don't grieve for me while I'm still here. Time enough for that in the future. Hopefully the far future." He had always been the one to say, "Don't worry about something until there's something to worry about." And now I could see his worry. Even before this, we had agreed that if something happened to either one of us, the other one must try to carry on as well as possible, even if we didn't feel like it, for our kids' sake. Well, they were not kids anymore. They were all young men.

I asked Bruce, "How are we going to get through this?" and he said, "One day at a time Nic, we'll get through one day at a time. We'll just put one foot in front of the other, and go day by day." And that's what we did. We found a saying that we liked and continued to remind each other, "Look through the windshield, not the rearview mirror."

Bruce is the love of my life and I've been with him for 27 years. He was married before and had two awesome sons, Daniel and Steven. We got together in 1985, not long after his marriage had ended. We had actually known each other since grade 8! I remember thinking he was a hunk in high school. Since he swore he was never getting married again, it took us 11 years to get tie the knot. We just celebrated our 16th wedding anniversary, but our 27th year together.

Dan and Steve don't live near us anymore. Steve is an AVN technician in the Royal Canadian Air Force and lives in Trenton with his fiancée, Oceana, and her mom, Annabelle. Dan is a police officer and lives with his wife, Sheena, in Calgary. We had just seen both of them at Dan's wedding in

Calgary. It was wonderful to have all of us together. By that time, I hadn't been feeling well for a while, but didn't say anything to them because this was Dan and Sheena's time. I spent that whole trip from Surrey to Calgary lying on my side with the seat of the van reclined. I was determined to go, though. They were upset to find out about my diagnosis, but continued thinking positively and loving me from afar.

I told our eighteen-year old son, Luke, that I had "had cancer" but it had been removed and the chemo and radiation were to make sure all the cells were gone. That was true, but I didn't go into detail about the seriousness of it with him. From that point on, he had faith that I was healed or being healed. I think Luke knew a little of how scared I was, but because I am a paranoid mom, always worrying about him, he just thought I was being paranoid again. And I was good with that. I didn't want to cause him unnecessary worry.

My chemo started October 3, 2011 and radiation started during chemo, and ended December 14, 2011. I had four rounds of chemo with three days on, eighteen days off and 30 radiation treatments in 17 spots around my shorts area. I thought I would be hanging over the toilet 24/7 but I didn't even throw up until after the fourth round. They have good anti-nausea drugs now. The treatment was brutal, but I was willing to do anything to fight the cancer off, since they told me they were going for a "full cure." Apparently this type of cancer responds very well to chemo. I had a combination of Cisplatin and Etoposide and tried to think of it like Pac-Man eating up any cancer cells. For me, the worst part of treatment was the fatigue and the radiation burns.

Bruce and Luke were such blessings and did everything while I was going through treatment. Most days all I could do was lie in the recliner. I was blessed with friends and family who brought meals and sent cards and flowers. I felt so loved. My sister, Adda, came over from Vancouver Island quite often and that was wonderful! She was with me for my first appointment at the Fraser Valley Cancer Centre. I remember they were checking for metastases and the doctor left the room to go get my scan results. I had a look of horror on my face, I'm sure, and Adda just grabbed me and hugged me and prayed that the scans would be clear. We stood like that and she prayed the whole time until the doctor came back. When she walked in, she didn't look at me at first and that scared the daylights out of me. Then she said they hadn't seen any signs of spreading. What a huge relief.

I had a "chemo buddy" with me every session. My buddy would drive me there, stay with me and talk to me all during chemo then get me back home and settled in. I felt very lucky to have these people in my life. I felt an amazing outpouring of love from my friends and family.

After treatment they said I was in remission, but not considered cured for two years. Funny thing with cancer, actually, not so funny, is that once you've had it, there is a fear of recurrence that is hard to forget. And with this type of cancer that is heightened.

Living as a survivor of this type of cancer has its challenges because you're always afraid it will come back. To make it worse, my oncologist had no plans for follow-up scans. She said I would feel a recurrence before it would be picked up on a scan. But one of my symptoms was fatigue and that was still there.

This is actually my second go round with cancer. The first time was 16 years ago when I had a lump on the floor of my mouth. My dentist had been examining my mouth and pressed on something and asked, "Does that hurt?" I said, "No." and he never said anything else about it. Of course, when I left the dentist, I had to feel in there to see what he was talking about and there was a lump. I wasn't too concerned, but then I was walking down the hallway at home and I heard a voice say, "You have cancer." I wasn't even thinking about the lump. I stopped, went into the bathroom and looked at myself in the mirror like I must be crazy. Then I heard the voice again, "You have cancer." That was pretty freaky. I was not saying it. It was someone else.

The doctor said it was a cyst in my salivary gland, but after hearing that voice, I was scared. I asked to see a specialist and was sent to an ear, nose and throat specialist then to an oral surgeon who did a biopsy. The biopsy got squished, but they suspected it might be cancerous. So I was sent to the top head and neck cancer surgeon in Vancouver. He supposedly removed the lump, but when I gingerly felt around in my mouth a few weeks after the surgery, I could still feel the same lump!

What the Hell? My doctor told me to go right back to the surgeon and the surgeon was actually annoyed at me for telling him the lump was still there. He told me this was a new lump, but I knew it was the one I had been feeling all along. He removed it and found it was adenocarcinoma. He told me the first lump he took out wasn't cancer, so I was relieved until I felt the lump was still there. I was very lucky that I pushed. They took out the left floor of my mouth and slit my neck to get lymph nodes out to check for spread. Luckily, I had gotten back in time so it hadn't spread and I didn't have to have chemo or radiation. But by then I looked like the bride of Frankenstein with staples along about eight inches on the side of my neck.

Regarding the Small Cell Cancer, I have now been in remission for 8 months. (Just over 12 if you count from when the lump was taken out.) It is very hard to live in fear of the cancer returning. I try to push the thoughts away, but they do come back. The little you can find on the Internet is just plain scary with a poor prognosis, no studies and just very little information on it.

I found the Small/Large Cell Cervical Cancer support group on Facebook through Angela Van Treuren. I was having another sleepless night and started Googling. Angela's blog popped up and she said she had small cell neuroendocrine. She led me to the group and the support the girls share is remarkable. They care for you, pray for you, answer any questions you have about treatment, symptoms, tests, etc. It really has been a Godsend to be able to ask someone your questions and get real, honest answers and several opinions. Many of the sisters are in remission, and many are in the heat of the battle. Some of the ladies pray, some don't. Many of these ladies will do anything they can to help you, and when you are ill or in treatment, they check up on you. There are ladies here from all over the world. We share information, love, healing, positive thoughts, and most importantly, hope. Here is one of my recent posts:

"Melanie and Colleen started this group. Angela Van Treuren has done a lot too. Honestly, I would be in a lot worse place emotionally if it weren't for you all and this group. The love and support we give and get here, well, there are no words. Maybe this was part of God's plan for you. I can't even imagine how many people you have helped. Yes, some have passed, but their final days were brighter and made easier because of your efforts and the love and support of the ladies here. Until I found this group, I felt so alone. Even though I had my wonderful family, no one really understood what I was going through until I met you guys. I know you three, and hopefully all of us, will touch many, many more lives in the months and years to come. :) Thank you for everything, ladies. And may you be blessed many times over for all the blessings you have given others. :) I love you."

There is a very nice doctor on the site, Dr. Michael Frumovitz, who we call Dr. F. He is a gynecological oncologist who works at MD Anderson in Texas. He answers people's questions and is starting to do extensive research on small and large cell neuroendocrine cancers. He told me he scans people every three or four months for the first few years and I am now using that note to try and get my oncologist to do that.

Some of my anxiety comes from the fact that they don't plan to scan me unless I feel something is wrong. But I can't tell if the fatigue, which is still quite bad, is a side effect from treatment, or from cancer, or from menopause, which I was rudely put into during radiation treatments. It was bugging me that the only other person who I have found with this type of cancer in her rectum just died this past July. She had gone into remission and then it came roaring back. But recently, I talked to someone whose mom had it in the same place years ago and she's now in her 80s. Some of the ladies, (we actually call each other sisters), wrote me their stories of having recurrences and how catching them early probably saved their lives. I put their information in a letter to my oncologist and she has now agreed to scan and ultrasound me every six months! Here's my post to the group about the ladies who helped me.

"I have to send you out my little piece of good news and I'm not going to apologize. In the long run, three of my sisters, Colleen Marlett, Angela Good Depriest, and Mona Wike gave me their stories of surviving recurrences and how their regular scans helped catch it early. I sent them as part of my plea to my oncologist and I am now seeing her Monday. Hoping she is going to change her mind. If she does, these 3 sisters may just save my life one day. Their stories can give us all hope. Mona has had two recurrences and been cancer free since fall 2008. Angela had spread to her lungs and lymph nodes in her abdomen and is 2 1/2 years cancer free now. Colleen had a recurrence after 18 months of remission and in September will be 3 years cancer free! To all of you sisters battling...have hope and NEGU (never, ever give up)."

I now have a "survivorship plan". My GP is going to do several blood tests, every three months, to keep an eye on several things. I am seeing a naturopath to help rebuild my immune system and prevent a recurrence. And now the oncologist is keeping a better eye out for it. All these things have helped calm me down a lot. I do a lot of positive self talk and thank God for curing me. Just have to keep pushing back the fear until I get more time under my belt. With this group of ladies cheering me on, I hope to get years and years of remission under my belt.

If you can learn anything from me, it is to TAKE CONTROL OF YOUR HEALTH!!!

If you think something is wrong and you're not getting answers, push harder or go to another doctor until they find out what is wrong with you. The doctors can't feel inside your body like you can. I had to push the whole way. And if I hadn't, I probably wouldn't be here to tell my story.

ACT if you feel something is wrong. Listen to that gut instinct, voice in your ear, message from God or whatever you want to call it. You must listen to your body and if you know something is not normal, get it checked and push until you have an answer. I believe that saved my life more than once now.

And my last piece of advice I will leave you with is this: never ever smoke. And if you do, throw your cigarettes away right now before something bad happens to you!! I still struggle with this addiction.

Nicole Atchison

**An update from Nicole was posted to the Small/Large Cell Facebook page on May 7, 2013, right before the completion of this book. This is what it said:

May 7, 2013

"My heart is so full of all my sisters and the supporters of this group. I've been writing my thoughts to you in my head for days, since I had the great pleasure and gift of actually meeting some of you in Vegas. When I was first diagnosed in Sept. 2011, I was desperately trying to find someone, anyone who had this rare, aggressive bitch cancer that had a poor prognosis and was known to be sneaky, and come

back. Of COURSE I Googled it. I'm just like that. I have a strong need to know and do my research when I want to know about something. The bit I did find out scared the crap out of me! I started a Facebook group called "Small Cell Neuroendocrine Carcinoma" and the only people who have EVER joined were Brandon Cagle, Jamie Cagle's (RIP SBJ) husband and one of their friends. Even to this day no one else has asked to join!

Finally, I ended up finding Angela Flick's blog, got in touch with her and she suggested that I join the group. I wasn't sure you would accept an "anal" sister, but you DID accept me, with open arms! Before our group, I would never have imagined that you could love someone so much without ever meeting them in person. I mean we're talking about a Facebook group! COME ON! At first I felt removed, being anal and all. My sign is zebra (for rare cancers), and I can't take part in the studies because mine was not in the cervix. But you ladies wrapped your arms around me and took me in. When I was freaking about an MRI, you were there, calming me down, cheering me on, sending prayers and hugs. Same thing with scan time, which we all face with hope and dread. After treatments, my oncologist wasn't even planning to ever scan me unless I had symptoms. But so many of you were being scanned on a regular basis. She told me I would have symptoms if it came back in the same area, before it would show up on a CT. She said if it came back anywhere else it was incurable anyway. But then Colleen Marlett, Mona Wike, and Angela Good Depriest sent me their stories and Dr. Michael Frumovitz told me he does it and he would recommend it. I put all that together in a letter, which resulted in me getting scanned. She was going to scan one time and ultrasound the next time (every three months). I tried for PET/CT but we only have two in the province of BC, and my oncologist felt that it was not needed. These past few months, 2 CTs showed my lymph nodes growing about a mm. a month, so finally a PET/CT was ordered. And low and behold, I lit up from my groin to my esophagus in the lymph nodes. The SUV level in some was 2.9 and 3.5 but the abdominal nodes lit up to 10! Some light ups might be from radiation damage.

The biopsy they did on the abdominal node was positive for small cell. I don't feel that all the nodes that lit up are from small cell. I had an abscessed tooth and a kidney stone going on at the time of PET. I was not expecting to find out the biopsy results until Monday, when I came home from Vegas, at the earliest. But I had emailed Dr. Le and said if she found out early, could she call me while I was in Vegas since I would be with some of you survivors, warriors and supporters. She was conferencing my case the Tuesday before I left for Vegas on Wednesday. The biopsy had just been done on Friday, so I wasn't expecting results on Tuesday! I thought she was calling about the conference and how to biopsy under my arm since nodes weren't swollen, they only lit up.

When she told that the biopsy was back and it was small cell and she said "incurable", I was devastated and heartbroken. And here is my nineteen year-old son, Lucas, staring at me in the store parking lot, shocked by what he was hearing by my answers to the doctor. We were sooo going with the infection! But, you ladies started correcting me right away when I used the word incurable. Many of you wrote personal notes on the site, reminding me of your stories of recurrences and now being cancer free, some for 5, 6, 7 years. To be going to Vegas to meet some of you the day after I had found out, well, it was an incredible, life-altering gift! And I do mean gift, since I couldn't afford to go and my flight and hotel were paid for by generous supporters and sisters. Someone named Julie Hewett paid for my flight and she's not even in the group! Sandy Hanson Ruth made and sold teal SMILE shirts to raise funds. So many people contributed to get I think eight of us there who could not have gone otherwise. Melanie Cummings, the whole trip just would not have happened without you and Colleen Marlett. We would have none of this if it weren't for you both and your tireless (sometimes not so tireless) work for our group! I am so grateful for you both, for the sisters and for Dr. Michael Frumovitz, who helped me get my doctor to scan me. You have saved and/or prolonged my life by helping me do that! I came home from Vegas with my warrior pants on and all the hope in the world that I can kick this bitch back into remission! I AM going to kick it into remission. Cancer, you have been given your eviction notice, now pack up and getouttahere!!! Together we are quite a force. A MOVEMENT! And here is how awesome Dr. Frumovitz and Dr. Jen Burzawa are. They flew from Texas to Vegas for one night, just to have dinner with us! I couldn't believe that! Amazeballs! I love each and every one of you and I always pray for your healing, comfort and a cure. I am more grateful to you than I can ever put into words (although I'm just tried :)) xox"

Debbie White's Story:

Deborah Jane White

My SCCC Story

I was diagnosed with Small Cell Neuroendocrine Carcinoma of the Cervix in August of 2010. But first, a little bit about me. Ken and I married young. We were 17 and we had both of our children by 19. We have 2 children, Mike and Crystal. We have 2 grandchildren, Tyler and Kacey. We have a large extended family that lives in our area. We are blessed. I was working a fulltime job when life took a turn. I was on my feet most of the time at work. One day I woke up with a backache. I told myself that I needed to get to the chiropractor; I must be out of alignment or something. I made my appointment and had x-rays done. The chiropractor told me that I would need to come in 3 days a week to get my back in order. I went to see him for three weeks. The pain started to come around to the front of my stomach and I told myself that it must be nerves getting pinched because of the adjustments. I continued to go to work, although I was in such pain. For example, after my adjustments with the chiropractor, I would lie there on the table and cry. They would put an ice pack on my back and I would stay until I could get myself together. My husband would drive me to work and I would lay the seat back to give me some relief because it hurt more to sit up straight. I would go into the conference room on my breaks and lie on the floor on my stomach, hoping the pain would cease. It got to where I could not sit in a chair because of the pain. Why didn't I go to the doctor sooner? I never dreamed that it could be cancer or anything bad.

After 3 weeks of this my husband took me to the emergency room. I must say I was the one who didn't think I needed to go sooner. They thought, at first, I was having some problem with my colon. They did an x-ray and a doctor came in and said, "You are messed up, girl. You have a mass of some sort." We were in shock. Soon after that, they came in with a shot of Dilauded and I remember sinking back onto the bed. Finally something for the pain, I was able to relax. I was taken to surgery for a biopsy right away. I was told I had a 7 cm tumor on my cervix. What? They told me I had cancer but they didn't know what kind. They sent the biopsy to L.A. and said it would take about a week for the results to come back. I was sent home with a pain patch to wait for results.

The news was a shock to my whole family. My friend since the 4th grade, Donna, came from Bakersfield as soon as she got the news. She was there to help with whatever my family needed. I was very uncomfortable that week, to say the least. I knew I had lots of people praying for me. My sister-in-law, Donna, had put me on the prayer list at church. During my most miserable time at home the ladies, my friends, came into my bedroom, laid hands on me and prayed for me while Linda and Brandi sang and played worship music. This was a beautiful example of how we should come together when someone is hurting and in need of prayer. Teresa, a family friend, came over the next day to give me a massage. When I was getting my massage she asked me if my ankle was hurt because it was swollen. I hadn't noticed until then. Indeed, it was swollen, but why? It became hard to go to the bathroom and I went to my family doctor for help but was sent home. I was just waiting for the biopsy results to come back. I remember taking Ambien at 4:00 PM. I just wanted to sleep. I woke up about 2:00 AM and knew I needed to get to the hospital. Ken put the back seat down and I lay in the back of the Bronco. I couldn't sit. We went back to the emergency room. The urologist came in and told us that my kidneys were in trouble. I was becoming septic and needed stents right away. They sent me to surgery and put in the stents between the kidneys and bladder, and inserted a catheter. My leg turned into an elephant leg. It was huge and looked like it could burst. It was lymphedema. The tumor was cutting off something to my leg. I was admitted to the hospital and the results came a few days after that.

Dr. Figueroa from Solace Cancer Care came to my room and told me about the cancer. He said it was a rare form of cancer called Small Cell Neuroendocrine Carcinoma of the Cervix. He said that I hadn't done anything wrong, and that it was as if I was driving down the highway and got sideswiped by a random car. I was not a candidate for a hysterectomy because of the size and type of cancer. He said that I had a sack of fluid in my abdomen and lymph nodes were inflamed. Doing surgery would most definitely let it spread. He told me that I would do my first round of chemotherapy in the hospital. I asked him to pray about my treatment before giving it to me and he assured me that he would. That comforted me. I remember my husband getting into the hospital bed with me late at night and holding me tight. I know he was praying for God not to take me away.

It had been almost 2 years since my last PAP smear. I have never had an irregular PAP in my life and my last one was clear also. I had always had regular periods, but had started to bleed irregularly. I had been having irregular bleeding for a while and the doctor assured me it was just perimenopause. During those 21 months, I had to wear a pad for bleeding every day. Sometimes it was worse than others and I had a few episodes of very heavy bleeding and clotting.

I knew in my heart I was in a bad situation. You realize that this life is so short. I'm not done yet! What about my dreams? My children and grandchildren need me! I didn't want to know what stage my cancer was. The doctor never told me and I didn't ask. Some family members thought I should know, but I didn't think so. I needed to focus on getting better. I didn't want anything that I heard to interfere with my faith that I would get better. It was during this time that Stacey was on the computer and found the SCCC Sisters Facebook page. There were only 12 girls on it, at that time. They let Stacey join as a supporter. It was through her that I would get information about the disease and the sisters. I never went online to look up small cell cancer. I suppose I was protecting myself.

I spent about 3 weeks in the hospital. My husband, son and daughter were all working long hours and would come to see me at night. My mom was always there to support me, but this was very hard on her. My daughter-in-law, Stacey, would stay with me at night and push my pain button every few hours so I could sleep. How great is that? She would bring Tyler (3 ½) and Kacey (6 months), my grandkids, to see me, and they would get into bed with me and watch America's Funniest Home Videos. Tyler would just crack up! He still remembers this and mentions it sometimes. I would think that, more than anything, I want to be alive for the grandchildren I have, and the ones yet to come. Crystal was 30 years old, with no children yet. My grandchildren had lived in my heart way before they were ever born and they are such a blessing!

My family had been planning my 50th birthday party but I would be turning 50 in the hospital now. My mom and kids got me ready to go to my party in the hospital cafeteria. I know I must have been a sight to my family and friends. I limped in with my walker and elephant leg. Stacey had wrapped my urine bag with birthday paper because I didn't want anyone to see it. I was greeted with lots of love and well wishes, red velvet cake and balloons. The party was short but sweet, as I couldn't sit or get comfortable.

I got through my first round of Cisplatin and Etoposide, my chemo cocktail. I was not good at staying on top of the nausea and was so sick! Dr. Fig had only told me that we would do a round of chemo in the hospital and then 21 days later, we would do another. We would then do a CT scan and check the status of my cancer. I'm finding that it is almost like having a baby. You forget about all that you went through after a while. When you are with others who are going through the same thing, or you are trying to recount all that happened to write it down, it all comes back to you and you remember. I remember being very weak and sick, hoping I could get outdoors and feel good and exercise. I remember that the bathroom was a big issue for me. I was so scared to get my catheter taken out. You know you can't leave the hospital until you go "beep" and that was horrible. I won't go into details, but I did go home and continued my treatment. My family would bring me food that I would have normally loved and I wouldn't be able to eat. My sister-in-law, Andi, would make her famous nut bread. My mom was sure I would be able to eat that, but, no. Nothing tasted good! Campbell's Vegetable Beef Soup was the only thing that sustained me.

After round 2 of chemo I went for my CT scan. I had faith that I would get good news and would be done with treatment. Stacey would tell me, "No, you are not done with treatment." And I would say, "Yes I am!" After all, I could sit normally now and knew the tumor was going or gone. My mom, Ken and Stacey went with me to see Dr. Fig and get the results. Dr. Fig came into the room and realized that he had not looked at my CT scan results yet. He said he would be back and left the room. He was gone about 15 long minutes. He came back into the room and said, "Well, we don't see anything." I said, "Halleluiah! Thank you, Jesus!" My mom said, "What? Ok, her tumor was the size of a baseball. Is it a golf ball, or marble size now?" The doctor said, "We can't see anything. No tumor!" I said, "Yeah!" Dr. Fig proceeded to tell me that he was scheduling the next round of treatment. Tears were rolling down my face and I was asking, "Why? It's gone!" The doctor said, "Look at me." He was looking straight into my face and reminded me of the kind of cancer this was and what we were dealing with. He said, "I will bring you to the brink of death to kill this cancer. If one little cancer cell gets away and hides behind your liver or somewhere, It will come back to get you." He wanted me to do a total of 7 rounds of chemo. Two rounds were hard for me. How would I do 7? He also told me to make an appointment with Dr. Pereira, the radiation oncologist. "Poop!" That's all I had to say! Stacey said, "I told you." She had been following the sisters on Facebook and knew treatment wouldn't be easy.

At this point I knew for sure I had the victory over this cancer! Jesus was with me and I had to fight. All I could say was, "One day at a time." I could not look at the big picture. It was just too overwhelming. Just put one foot in front of the other. Look at what is right in front of you and deal with that. At some point you will get to the end of it. That's what I did.

I only made it through 4 rounds of Cisplatin/Etoposide

because I started having signs of nerve damage, such as numb feet and hands and ringing in my ears. For round 5 we switched to Carboplatin. I had to have blood transfusions and platelets after rounds 3, 4 and 5. Dehydration was also a problem for me and I would have to go in for IV fluids often. With all of the signs my body was giving, Dr. Fig put a stop to chemo after the 5th round.

I had my radiation during November of 2010. While getting prepped for the radiation treatments, I received my first tattoos. Three little black dots, one below the belly button and one on each hip, were permanently marked on my body. These would be guides for the red beam of light. They also made a mold of my body. I would lie in it each time I received radiation. You have to lie very still to make sure the beams hit the same spots each time. I had 25 treatments. I will always remember Dean. He was working in radiation and was so kind to me. They all were very supportive. They would get me all set up on the table and would shut the big, metal door behind them. They would go behind the glass and computer to start the machine that would move around my body and shoot red beams into me. I can tell you that, as soon as that door shut, my eyes were closed and I was with God. I would count my blessings, Thank Him for everything in my life. Things past, things present, and things to come. This is what I did every time! Sometimes it was like being transported back into a wonderful memory of when my kids were little. 20 minutes would seem like 3 minutes. This is how I got through it. I did not want to focus on the radiation except how it would contribute to my healing!

When I was told I would have to do internal radiation also, I was not a happy camper. I was scared! I was told they would clamp metal barbells to my cervix at the hospital and then transport me back to Solace Cancer Care to administer the radiation vaginally, directly onto the cervix. Then Dr. Pereira would remove them. Yuck, this was the worst thing. I had this done two times.

I went in for my vaginal check with Dr Pereira. She was looking at my cervix and said, "Oh my!" That made me nervous and I was wondering what had happened. She said, "That is the best looking cervix! It's pink and you can barely see a light purple spot where the tumor was." I said, "Praise the Lord!" My husband and I tease now and say that I have the best looking cervix in town.

My daughter, Crystal, found out she was pregnant on Christmas Morning of that year. God's timing is perfect. What a gift. We were at my mom's for Christmas Dinner that night and she was at the stove, cooking. I said, "Should we tell her?" Mom just started crying and saying, "No! No! No!" The first thing she thought was that something was wrong with me and she couldn't bear to hear it. That's when I knew the cancer was actually harder on her than it was on me. Crystal gave birth to Lukas on August 21, 2011. And I was there!

My scans had been clear for two years and Stacey and Donna told me that they heard about another girl in our area, diagnosed with the same thing. Her name is Stephanie Walker Stika. I went to her benefit and met her. My doctor had told her that she had 3 months to live and shouldn't bother with treatment. That's crazy! There is always hope! You must fight! Her story is for her to tell, but at my next appointment, I finally asked about my stage of cancer. He told me it was 4a. I needed to tell Stephanie. She can get through this too! I was blessed a few weeks ago and was able to go to Las Vegas with Stephanie. We got to be with the other SCCC sisters. What a wonderful group of women. I'm telling you good things come out of bad situations all the time. That is how God works. We had a great time together.

I can tell you that I do consider myself to be healed. Cancer free! I choose to walk in that truth. That does not mean there aren't struggles. Fear tries to creep in and I have to push it out. An unexpected pain here or there can bring a panic. When I told my husband I needed to write my story for the book, he said, "I know you are going to write about how you were healed, but what about the other women who prayed just as hard and died?" He has a good point. It breaks my heart that we lose so many to this disease. I think about the conversation we had with Pixie and Kerri at the pool in Las Vegas. They lost Meredith in 2007. The pain in their eyes, as they spoke of the daughter and sister they lost, was as if it had happened yesterday. Kerri told me about how she begged God to heal her sister. She just wanted to see her live her life! I know she is alive.

I obviously don't have all of the answers, but I do know that God loves us. He is love. We sometimes think that this life on Earth is the only life. This is only the beginning. After this life, no matter how long or how short, comes Eternity. Our tents (bodies) wear out and then we have to move out. These bodies are not permanent. The question is, do we believe God? Or man? John 3:16 and 17 Red letters "For God so loved the world that He gave His only begotten Son, that whoever believes in Him should not perish but have everlasting life." 17 "For God did not send His Son into the world to condemn the world, but that the world through Him might be saved." He has already chosen you. He is waiting at the door of your heart for you to open and let

Him in.

I want to thank all of my friends and family for their support. I was not able to acknowledge everyone in this short story, but I remember all that you have done for me.

Remember to live while you're alive! I intend to. Love you all.

Our next story is from a women that found us by accident. Although we do not know if she ever had SCCC or LCCC, as she has since left the group to move on from "cancer land", and never clearly mentions it in her story, we are sure she faced a very scary diagnosis for her. SCCC and LCCC is usually treated with chemo, coupled with radiation and sometimes the combination of surgery as well. These treatments may vary, but it is never common practice for SCCC or LCCC, at any stage, to be treated with a LEEP procedure. Any diagnosis of cancer is scary even the pre-cancerous stages and Lisa's story could be any woman's in the world. We thank her for sharing it with us.

Lisa Beimer's Story:

Lisa Nicole Beimers, age 33, Kentwood, Michigan

My story actually started before my diagnosis was made. You see, four years prior to my diagnosis in 2012, my husband was killed in a car accident by someone texting and driving. That event left me alone, raising three amazing boys all by myself. It isn't an easy job by any means, but I never thought for a single second that there could be something growing inside of me that could kill me.

The last checkup I had was right after my husband passed away. I wanted to make sure to get as many checkups for the boys and me before my husband's health insurance ran out. After that, the thought of getting a checkup crossed my mind, but I never took it seriously. I always thought that nothing would ever happen to me so it just could wait one more year. Little did I know that without a checkup, that one more year could've been my last.

I finally got accepted to Medicaid in August of 2011. I should have gone straight to the doctor to get my checkup, but I didn't. I still thought I was invincible. I was starting to get pain in my mid-section, but every time I went to the ER to have it checked, they had some kind of simple explanation for the pain. They never thought to get me into the stirrups to see if there could be a problem "in there." You should have heard their explanations: gall bladder, B.V., acid reflux, and the best one, intestinal infection. The outcome was always the same: send me home with some sort of medication. I was beginning to think that I was going to live in pain for the rest of my life.

Over the months the pain got worse. Then my period started doing some crazy stuff like showing up late and discharging extra mucus all month long. Most annoying of all was the change in the duration. One month I would have it for three days, it would stop for one day, and then continue for four more days. The next month it would show up a week early and last for two days. In my mind I thought it was because of the stress of losing a husband and learning to be a single parent. As I look back I realize I should have run to the doctor to get that long overdue *checkup. But hey, it will never happen to me, right?*

March 19th 2012 was the official start to one of the scariest events in my life. That is when I finally went to get my "girly" checkup for the first time in three years. The doctor visit was as normal as could be, right down to the paper gown. When I sat up and my doctor was washing his hands, he asked me if I had ever had an abnormal PAP smear. I told him, "No," and chuckled a little bit then asked, "Why?" He just told me I probably have nothing to worry about, but since I am sexually active, I should see him every year. I just took it as no big deal and went home.

My doctor's office has one of those systems where you can look at your chart anytime. About four days later, I looked at the chart and noticed that my PAP was indeed abnormal. I was concerned but was still in denial that anything could be wrong. I told my mom and my sister about what was going on and they were also assuring me that everything was going to be okay. My doctor called me into his office the next day and said that he was referring me to an OB/GYN surgeon. Again, I thought that was okay since I wanted to get my tubes tied anyway. It was like hitting two birds with one stone.

It is amazing how fast everything goes when the doctors think something is wrong. It is also amazing that they try to convince you that everything will be okay, when in reality, they have no idea if that's the case. I know they do that to keep you calm and to avoid lawsuits, but it doesn't help when you receive the news that will change everything in your life. I went to the surgeon and had to have a biopsy, which didn't hurt as much as I thought it would. Yes, it was uncomfortable, but no worse than getting a tattoo or giving birth. When he was done, the surgeon told me we would have the results in a few days, and then gave me the same old, "Don't worry. I'm sure everything will be fine."

On Monday morning I was sitting at the computer, like I do every morning, drinking my coffee and checking Facebook. I decided to check my chart online again and I saw it. I saw it right there in black and white print. I, Lisa Nicole Beimers, have cervical cancer?! I froze. I even blinked and rubbed my eyes. Was I reading this right? I am only 33 years old. I ran straight to the phone and called my doctor. Of course he and his nurse were busy and would have to call me back. Call me back?! I have something in me that will kill me and you are too busy to answer my call? At this point I really didn't care about anything else he had going on.

I texted my older sister next. I just couldn't get myself to say it out loud. She, of course, called me right back. That was the first time I could hear fear in her voice. She started asking me the same questions I was wondering. I explained that I still did not know how bad it was or any other details, so I needed to wait until I heard from the doctor. My sister then asked me if I had told Mom. Of course I had not told Mom, she was at work. My sister gave me Mom's work number and told me I should call and tell her. The truth is, I couldn't tell her. How can you tell the woman that gave birth to you whom you love so much that you have cancer? My mom had already lost her mom to lung cancer and her brother had just passed of lung cancer, not even 5 months earlier. Now she'll have to hear that her youngest daughter has cancer, too?

I finally asked my sister to tell my mom the news and,

thankfully, she was willing to do so. While I was waiting for her to call me back, my doctor's nurse called. She told me that my cancer was early stage 1 and the doctor wanted to do a LEEP procedure first, before talking about doing anything radical. The LEEP procedure had an 85% chance of successfully removing the cancer. I told my nurse that 85% chance is just not going to cut it because that still leaves a 15% chance of recurrence. I, personally, did not like those odds, so I told her I wanted a hysterectomy and I would not take, "no" for an answer. She told me that she would let the doctor know and I should discuss it with him when I come in for my appointment the next day.

When I got off from the phone I lost it. I could not stop shaking and crying. The thing is, I wasn't feeling sorry for myself. I was more worried about my boys, my mom, my dad, and my sisters. Most of all, I was scared that my boys would lose their mom after already losing their dad. I knew stage 1 was good news and had good outcomes, but fear can take away every ounce of hope you may still have.

When my older sister called me back, I told her it was stage 1 and I could hear the relief in her voice. She felt the same way I did. My uterus just had to go. With our family's history of cancer, we were not going to let that monster take another one of us. We were going to beat it. One of the hardest things for me was talking to my mom about it. Even though she had her brave face on, I could tell that her heart was breaking with fear.

The next day I went to the doctor and I started to plead my case to him. I do not remember much, but I do remember giving him all of the information about our family's history of cancer. I have already mentioned my grandma and uncle, but there were many more. My cousin with a brain tumor, aunts with ovarian cancer, etc. It seems like every kind of cancer has been in our family. That is why I knew with all of my heart that cancer is hereditary, even though my doctor said their cancers had nothing to do with mine. Thankfully, he told me that he would do the surgery for me, and all we needed to do was get Medicaid's permission to do so. But we needed to get it done as soon as possible because my type of cancer can be aggressive and spread quickly. The hysterectomy was scheduled for two weeks from that day.

I left the office that day, thankful that they had agreed to perform the hysterectomy, but also concerned about how I would get everything done by myself. Not only did I have to make sure I had a ride to and from the hospital, I also had to make sure my life insurance and my will were in order and find a place for the kids to stay during surgery and recovery. I even went as far as to write letters to my boys, my parents, my sisters and the boys' Godparents, just in case something went wrong with the surgery.

I tried to show everyone that I was not scared, even though I was trembling inside. What if this thing is going to kill me? My boys just lost their dad, how could God do that to them? I had so many questions and concerns, and everyone around me was pretending to be brave, just as I was.

One day I decided to type "cervical cancer" in the search bar on Facebook. The first site I saw was an open site. I quickly dismissed that group because I wanted a place to post my feelings that would be private and hidden from my general Facebook friends. In my second search attempt, I found the SCCC/LCCC Sisterhood. The minute I read about this page I had no doubt it was where I belonged. I typed a little bit of information about myself and waited to see if I was going to be accepted into the "invite only" group. Within seconds I was welcomed into the sisterhood and lovingly introduced to the whole group in a status post. I couldn't believe that these women, who had no idea who I was, were so happy to have me there. At first I was too scared to post much of anything. Again, I wanted to seem strong. But after my first post, I realized that these women cared about me and wanted me to have all the information I needed to make informed decisions with my doctor. And guess what? The best part was they had the same feelings that I did. THEY UNDERSTOOD! That was something my friends and family couldn't do because, thankfully, they have never gone through this. I would not wish this cancer on anyone, not even my enemies

I told a few people I trusted at my church what was going on with my health, but I stressed that they could not say anything in front of my boys. I did not want them to know about it until they absolutely needed to. I also needed to get a handle on everything before I shared this information with them. I knew they would be just as, if not more, scared than I was.

The day I scheduled my surgery, my friend came over to visit. I sat down with him and told him everything that was going on. He said, "Oh, well, it was caught early. You will be fine" And then he started to whine and complain about his life. He was upset because I wasn't being my usual self and calming him down about his problems. But hey, I had just found out a monster was living in me. How was I supposed to act? As he was leaving my house, he told me that, even though I was studying to become a pastor, I would never make a good one because I didn't seem to care about other people's problems. I finally blew up and told him that I had cancer and the whole world didn't always revolve around him. I found out that he later badmouthed me to a mutual friend, so I blocked him from my phone and Facebook. That experience taught me that some people only wanted to be my friend when it was always about them, but Heaven forbid I had a problem in my life. Where were they when I needed them? Oh well. I had more important things on my mind.

The time between my diagnosis and my surgery flew by. I was truly blessed to have my kids' Godparents around to take care of them until I was able to get home from the hospital. Also, my church had a lineup of some wonderful ladies who planned to make meals for the kids and me for two weeks.

The next thing I knew, it was the night before the surgery. That was when the true fear kicked in. What if I didn't make it? Would this be the last time I'd see my boys? All these thoughts and fears raced through my mind. Of course, I did not sleep at all. When I did try to sleep I kept my bedroom light on, just like I did when I was scared at night as a child. I honestly didn't want to fall asleep. If there was a chance I was not going to make it, I surely did not want to spend my next few hours, minutes, and seconds asleep. Then my alarm went off and I knew my mom would be over to pick me up thirty minutes later. I went to the bathroom and smoked what would end up being my last cigarette, and took a shower. Then I went to all three of the boys' beds. I did not wake them but I kissed them each on the forehead and told them I loved them. I did not want to say goodbye, because goodbye had a whole new meaning to me.

My mother pulled into the hospital, and we went into the surgery center. I had walked past this room on numerous occasions, but had never given a thought to how the people inside were feeling. I was trying to be a big girl and to show my mom that I was a strong woman, but I really just wanted to hug her and never let go. We then went into the back room and they got me ready for the surgery. That was the longest forty-five minutes of my life. At that point I just wanted to get back there and get the monster out of me. The nurse came by and told me it was time then started to get the gurney into moving status. Then it happened. The tears started to roll out. I tried with all my might to hold them back, but I just couldn't. Just as they started to wheel me away, my mom yelled out, "I love you!" All I could do, while sobbing, was tell her that I loved her too. My mom doesn't say those words too often, so when she actually does, it makes them even more special to me.

I do not remember much of what was said as I was being wheeled to surgery. I know I kept cracking jokes to hide the fear I had inside of me. In my opinion, they need to put you to sleep before they take you to the operating room. It was a scary thing to see the inside of an operating room. It was a lot bigger and darker than I thought it would be. The last thing I remember was something being injected into the IV and it stinging a lot. My instinct was to pull it out, but I knew they would not do anything that would hurt me.

The next thing I remember is waking up, and at the same moment, asking, "Where is my mom?" They told me it would be a little while before I could see her. My body just wanted to go back to sleep, but I did my darnedest to stay awake. In my mind, I knew that if I saw my mom then everything was truly ok. Finally they brought me to my room, and yes, my mom was there, waiting for me, just as she had promised. I was ok! The rest of that day was very hazy. I do remember my sister and my niece coming to see me. My niece was so cute. She kept drawing pictures to make me feel better. People kept coming in and out of the room. It got to the point that I asked the nurse to please just let me sleep for a few hours. It wasn't only a few visitors, it was also the staff that kept on coming in to poke at me or check on me. All I wanted was some good rest.

Then, finally, at midnight it was time for me to get up and stand. It was as if they had asked me to climb Mt. Everest. There was so much pain! I thought I would never be able to stand. You take for granted being able to stand every day, that is, until you can barley do it at all. It felt like it took hours, but in reality it was only a few minutes. The nurses were very nice and rooted me on the whole time.

The next afternoon I got to go home. It was beyond wonderful being able to rest on my own couch. The horrible part was getting up to use the bathroom. Thank goodness I was able to use the back of the couch to pull myself up. Then, before I knew it, my boys were home. My eldest was amazing! He would make sure I had everything I needed, and even did the laundry and the dishes. I was one VERY proud mom. My boys banded together to take care of me, just like I had done with them so many times when they were ill. The only part my oldest hated was when I would drop the remote and he had to pick it up and give it back to me. I told him it was payback for all of the times he would drop a toy and have me pick it up when he was a baby.

Of course, there were the thoughtless people who ask and do the most stupid things when you are ill. All I wanted to say to them was, "Really?" But I didn't. I even had one person ask me to babysit her son about a week after my surgery. The thing that hurt the most was that my "best friend" at the time was downright mean to me. She had a hysterectomy about a year earlier and I thought she would have had compassion, but she did not. She even came to my house a couple of weeks after my surgery and told me to get my lazy butt up. ("Butt" was not the word she used.) I tried to tell her I had overdone it and I was in pain, but she just got nastier with her words. All I kept thinking was if she was a best friend, who needed enemies?

It also took me awhile to get my hormones under control. I would cry at a drop of a hat. Or, on the other hand, I would start getting utterly ticked off at every little thing that was going on.

My doctor decided that I did not need chemo or any additional treatments because the cancer had not spread (thank God) and it was in the VERY early stages. I would, however, need scans every six months for the first year, then every year for the next four years. This plan sometimes scares me, because I have seen many women have recurrences with this cancer. I keep telling myself, however, that everyone's situation is different. Just because Jane's cancer came back, that doesn't mean mine will.

That is another reason I love our sisterhood. I can tell them my fears and they will not degrade for them. I have tried to tell some other people that I am scared the cancer will come back, and they have actually told me I should just forget about it. It's done, right? They have no idea what it is like when I feel any pain now because I have a fear that it could be cancer. Or if I am extra tired then that could be cancer also. To everyone else, I am just being dramatic. But to me, it is real. Too real. I would love to go back to the days when, if I felt a pain, I could just assume it was something simple.

Since the surgery I have changed my life in so many ways. In fact, as of today it has been 132 days since my last cigarette. In the past it was very hard to quit smoking. Yes I knew the dangers, but I thought the same thing a lot of smokers think, "It won't happen to me." After having cancer once, I did not want to give it any more excuses to make itself at home in my body again, so I quit. And this time it's for good! I also eat as many foods that have anti-cancer properties as I can and I try to stay away from preservatives as well. The biggest change is that I exercise now. I am a plus size gal, and I always complained that I would never be fit again. The fact is I was too scared to try. Scared of what other people might think. Guess what? I do not care what others think anymore. I exercise at a minimum of 5 hours per week, and between you and me, I feel like a new woman. Cancer will always know that it is not welcome in my body ever again, because I fight like a girl!

This group of girls who are also sharing their stories with you in this book are AMAZING! I couldn't have gone through this without them. We bond together because we want the same thing, to bring awareness to this cancer. To let every woman know that it is VERY important to get your "box" checked regularly. If you put it off it may be too late if they do find something wrong. Take it from me and every lady in here, you do not want that to happen to you. Life is so very short as it is. Do not do anything to make it shorter. I pray every night for these ladies, and also for earlier detection. Not every woman is as lucky as I was to catch it early like I did. Check your box and keep on getting it checked! Do not blow off any symptoms! FIGHT LIKE A GIRL!

Joyce Crandall's Story:

My name is Joyce Crandall and I am now 1 woman in 1,000 who has been diagnosed with Small Cell Cervical Cancer.

How can that be, I wonder? I am no one special. Sure, I'm special to my son and to my three wonderfully rambunctious grandsons and to the rest of my family and friends. But basically I live a quiet, not-too-crazy life in northwest Illinois. I am 54 years old, average height, with highlighted blonde hair and hazel eyes. I have always watched what I eat and stayed in shape. Pretty normal, right? So how could I have this rare cancer? How am I now special? Especially considering that I don't really want to be.

Strangely I remember, not long before I had my first doctor's appointment with my gynecologist that would eventually lead to my "special" diagnosis, lying on my couch one day and suddenly taking a long, hard look at my body. I remember thinking how incredible and fragile a body is, and feeling overwhelmed by the love I have for my friends and family. I was proud of myself for having done the right things to keep myself healthy. I was feeling truly blessed.

My story is one of beginnings, as it has no end. I pray every day that will be the case for a very long time.

My journey really begins in early 2000, when I had an ovary burst. Following three days of lying in a hospital bed on morphine, my right ovary and fallopian tube were removed. Within five years of this procedure, I no longer had a period. Most women might have jumped at this prospect, but not I. To me, my period ceasing meant aging and I wasn't eager for anything connected with that. However, I am a firm believer that everything happens for a reason and, as I look back, I have to wonder if perhaps, further down my journey, this may be the thing I can look at as having helped to save my life, because the cancer was found early and was diagnosed at Stage 1b1.

I hadn't had this thought yet, however, when I was at work late in June 2012. I was in the restroom and noticed I was spotting, ever so lightly. Having not had a period in over seven years, I knew this was not a good sign. Returning to my office, I searched the Internet and the word "cancer" was everywhere I looked. To be honest, I had not been feeling quite right since the end of March. It seemed like every time I ate something I felt full and my stomach would bloat somewhat. Now that I was spotting too, I felt sick and scared. But I knew I had to be overreacting. Things like this only happen to other people. Having to wait a week to get in to see my doctor, I ignored the nurse's advice to stop searching the Internet. Sure, something was probably going on, but it would be some minor thing.

My internal voices were also external. My family and friends, my significant other and even my boss, who is a dear friend, everyone I knew kept telling me that everything was going to turn out just fine.

During my internal exam, my gynecologist made several comments that made me feel like he knew something wasn't quite right. Ordering an ultrasound, he told me the worst-case scenario was endocrine cancer, and stressed that it was most likely polyps. I could deal with polyps. That is what I was hanging my hopes on when I went in for my ultrasound a few days later. While doing the ultrasound the technician admitted to seeing a tumor but told me the wall was not thick enough for normal concern. So I left, holding onto the thought that it was just a fibroid tumor, perfectly treatable. My gynecologist scheduled a surgical biopsy for me and said he would do some exploratory while I was there. On July 11, 2012 I had that procedure. Later, I found out from my gynecologist that he knew that day it was cancer but had to wait for the official biopsies to come back. And when they did neither he nor the consulting oncologist could believe the type of cancer they were showing. Consequently, those biopsies were sent on to the Mayo Clinic for confirmation.

"Everything will be fine." Everyone was still saying it. I was saying it to myself. It had to be true. I told my significant other that I would be alright, driving to my appointment 35 minutes away. "Everything will be just fine," I said. My head said it was fine but my heart knew it wasn't. Looking back, I should have had someone come with me.

When my gynecologist walked into the room, his head slightly down, he said I had a tumor and that he got most of it while in surgery. But the sad news was that it was malignant and he went on to explain the limited information he was able to research on this type of cancer. I know my doctor, he most likely spent hours to find what he was able to find on SCCC. Wait. What did he say? Malignant? Did he really say that? At some point, when I started being able to listen to what he was saying again, there was even more to process. This was when the term

"Small Cell Cervical Cancer" (SCCC) became a part of my daily life, and when the 1 in 1,000 rarity of it would first be explained to me. And just like that, on July 17, 2012, "normal" me became "special."

He recommended a radical hysterectomy and requested that I meet with a local oncologist to get my plan started as quickly as possible, since this type of cancer is known to spread quickly. I was still holding it together. I was quite simply in shock! My gynecologist, who I have been seeing for a long time, assured me that I was more than a patient and that he would continue to research and to do everything he could to help me beat this. He kept telling me he couldn't believe how well I was taking this news. Well, Not really. But up until that point I hadn't broken down and was just trying not to lose it. I knew if one tear fell, I wouldn't be able to stop. Ever. He reached out to give me a hug and that was all it took. I said, "See what you made me do?" The tears started and I just saw my life ending.

In an odd twist, I had had a different appointment scheduled with my ear, nose and throat doctor to follow the appointment with my gynecologist. I had been struggling with sinus issues, had a CT scan performed on my sinuses, and I was now supposed to go and review those results. It was an appointment my doctor asked me to keep, if I was able, so the sinus scan could be reviewed for any possible tumors. But this doctor, the one who was just consoling me, had said "malignant" and "rare cancer." My sinus issues were now minor in my mind but I knew that he would not ask me to keep this appointment unless it was important.

I walked out, alone and crying. The world looked different somehow. I felt alone, scared and, as with anyone receiving a cancer diagnosis, I felt my life had come to an end way too early. I got into my car and made some calls I did not want to make to my son and daughter-in-law and my significant other. I could barely speak. In my mind I was calling to let them know I was diagnosed with cancer and was dying. I didn't have a lot of information for them since my doctor didn't have a lot for me on this rare kind. I told them as much as I knew and they just reassured me that we would fight this together, as they held back the tears. I then had to call my significant other. He was shocked, stunned and began to cry, while assuring me that we would get through this together.

I pulled myself together and drove 15 minutes down the road to my next appointment, crying all the way. In the waiting room, I huddled in the corner and continued to cry. Once I met with the ear, nose and throat doctor, we reviewed the scan and he said it was clear of tumors. He started giving me samples for my sinus symptoms but I had heard what I had come to find out. "My sinus issues are no longer my priority and, if I survive this, I will be back. But until then, I just can't focus on it," I said and left.

I had one more stop at the hospital to pick up the prep for my CT scan. I knew about the oral contrast I was going to have to drink from when I had had my colonoscopy a few years ago, that God awful stuff had made me miserable, throwing up every hour, all night long.

In a blessed twist of fate, a close friend of mine was on her way to the same hospital to see her newborn grandson. She met me in the lobby and we hugged and I cried some more. On my 45-minute drive back home, I called my boss and gave him the news. Stunned, he urged me to pull over.

Being supportive, he said he would come get me and, when I refused, he stayed on the phone with me for a long time. Once we hung up, the crying continued. When he called back to check on me, he said he, his wife and his young daughter wanted to come over and keep me company once I got home. The consistent support and encouragement of my family and friends really began in full-force that day.

Once I got home, I hugged my significant other and we just cried. Looking around my house, I saw everything differently. Sobbing non-stop, I started making some decisions about who I wanted to start giving my belongings to. Everything I saw conjured up happy memories...and pain. A Mickey Mouse trinket from Disneyworld, where I had visited with my family a few years prior. Such a happy, wonderful time and all I could think of was that I would never share Disneyworld again with my grandkids. My bed pillows that I bought from The Mirage in Las Vegas, a place I go to every September for my birthday. Again, I cried because it was now another place I would never see again. This went on all evening. My life was over. The next day I had to pull myself together and go to work, a very different person. Now I had cancer...and I didn't like it.

I called my direct reports into the conference room and told them my news so they didn't hear from anyone else. Telling my story over and over, it was one of the longest days of my life. My son and daughter-in-law had started doing research on the Internet and came across several articles, one of them written by a women who had survived SCCC. This article stood out and I read it several times. What had I found inspiring about her story? She lived!! But then I found that the website mentioned in this article was no longer there, which was devastating to me. I assumed there could be no reason other than the disease had taken her, for that website to no longer be there.

Knowing that I was looking for more information about this woman and others like her, one of my friends emailed me information on MD Anderson and a Facebook page for women with SCCC that included the woman in the article. I was so relieved to find this woman was alive. She is a survivor!! This was the beginning of me becoming a part of a very special group of women, each with a different story, but all with the same diagnosis and all who had a wealth of information. If you were scared, having a bad day, or just had a question, you could put it out there and within seconds, a flood of responses of support and answers would come your way. Some days on that site were very hard in the beginning, when I'd open it up to see the announcement that another "sister" had lost her battle. After processing the ups and downs of constant communication with these "sisters" I firmly believe that I am blessed to have found them.

On July 27th I met with the oncologist and that visit, along with the following two visits, were among the worst experiences I've ever encountered. Everyone in the waiting room looked like what I was certain my future was going to be. People so pale they looked like albinos, some with no hair, others so skinny and frail I am not sure how they were even walking. The doctor was extremely nice and young enough to be fresh out of school. He told me that, most likely, chemo was going to be part of the treatment. Later I found out that he really expected the Mayo Clinic to come back and say the diagnosis was wrong, he truly believed it was not SCCC. He went on to explain that, because this is so rare, there is no protocol for treatment and so we would be *following the treatment protocol for lung cancer. This was the beginning of many, many doctors telling me they were treating me as if I had lung cancer. And the beginning of my frustration over following a protocol for something I did not have.*

When the doctor followed up with me after he got the results back that confirmed SCCC, he went into detail about the rapid growth of my disease. My gynecologist agreed with him that I should have a radical hysterectomy as quickly as possible, then begin treatment as soon as I was released. Having already had a CT scan of my chest, he now also ordered a PET scan to see if the cancer had spread anywhere else. I felt like the tests would never end.

On July 22, I did my prep for the PET scan. But when I arrived at the hospital I was told that I was supposed to have done it that morning, so I had to do the prep all over again. I kept thinking that all of these tests surely must be some way of readying me for the horrible day that I would start chemo.

I went into the cold trailer that was attached to the hospital, to a very small room that smelled like chemicals, and my veins were injected with the radioactive material. I sat in a recliner for almost an hour in the dingy, cold room with the only brightness being orange signs: "WARNING RADIOACTIVE MATERIAL."

I could see out the window, through to the middle room, where the techs were on their computers, processing a PET scan in progress. I could also then look through their room, into the testing room, at the scanner and the patient in it. On some level this was nice because I knew where I was going, and where I was going was out of this horrible room.

The staff was just wonderful and when it came to my turn they patiently explained the process of the PET scan. I would be wheeled through once to take a picture and then sent fully back through six times, each time stopping for a picture that would take three minutes or so. So each time the machine stopped I counted 180 seconds in my head, it then moved and I counted again. This was the only way I could get through roughly a half hour without moving a single muscle. Otherwise they would have to do retakes, and I was determined that that was not going to happen. After each scan I took a breath and thought, 'one more picture closer to a cup of coffee.' I was in stress overload!

Shortly after this PET scan I went to see the radiation doctor for the first time, at a cancer center in Illinois. The staff was extremely nice and the center itself was beautiful and very comfortable. It was evident they really had the patient's needs in mind when they designed the center and they scheduled chemo appointments so a patient never had to wait in the waiting room. The radiation doctor went over what was, by now, becoming familiar territory. This was a fast-spreading, very rare cancer and so on. But what I had come to the center to hear from him was what came next. He said he would hesitate to do any type of preventative brain radiation or pelvic radiation, as he just could not justify the risks versus the benefits. He also mentioned that there is little to no data on this type of cancer and only found articles from 1998 and one from 2010, on which he partially based his findings. I left there feeling positive that, at least for my case, radiation was not warranted.

I followed this visit with another appointment at a different office with a senior oncologist and suddenly my buoyant feelings evaporated. From rude staff members to a two-

hour wait, the only thing that kept me waiting – impatiently - for the doctor was his reputation. Getting to my case, he said he was in favor of possibly getting another opinion because he was surprised the radiation doctor was not in favor of radiation. Now all of the positive feelings I had had at the outset of the day were completely gone. I did, however, determine that, despite an incredible reputation in its field, this office was not for me. I needed to put my faith and my trust and my life in the hands of a facility where I felt comfortable.

With my radical hysterectomy approaching on August 7th, I began my prep for the surgery on August 5th. The prep consisted of liquids all day and the following day, as well. The second day I started taking the pills instead of the liquid. I have a sensitive stomach and when I had to do this same prep for my colonoscopy a few years earlier, I threw up the whole night. Well, this time was no different and I did my best, but I cheated a little. Taking 4 horse pills every 15 minutes doesn't seem like it would be that difficult, but it was and I was sick and tired of it all, so I didn't take a few of the pills. I just couldn't do it.

I arrived at 5:30 AM on August 7th for my radical hysterectomy. <u>Fifteen</u> family members crowded my room and stayed with me until they took me into surgery. Just before, my gynecologist met with us and explained the procedure, warned everyone that my face would be swollen as I would be upside down while the surgery was being performed, and that it would take two to three hours. I admitted to him that I did cheat a bit on the prep and we all hoped for the best. Several hours later, I woke up in recovery and the first thing I remember is seeing my son and daughter-in-law. I then knew I was ok and I was alive.

I later found out that the surgery took five hours and I was in recovery for three-and-a-half hours before anyone was able to see me.

I settled in and began the very slow process of healing from such an invasive surgery. My projected few days in the hospital turned into seven days and, during that time, I was overwhelmed by the outpouring of love from my family and friends.

On my first day in the hospital, my whole family was with me for 12 hours and didn't leave until 6 PM, when I was so exhausted that I couldn't stay awake. However, three hours later, at 9 PM, I was wide awake, stuck in bed with an IV and Foley catheter, and I just felt a little lost. My good friend, who lived 10 minutes away, sent me her nightly happy text message. Through a few more text messages, she sensed that I was in need of a friend. When I typed "good night" to her, she threw her shoes on and came over and spent the next two hours with me until well after 11 PM. Her kindness really got me through that first night and it hasn't slowed down at all. My boss arrived the morning after surgery with flowers in hand. My significant other spent the night. My family was there every day, all day. My brother took the 1 ½ hour train ride out just to spend a few hours in the evening with me on the days he couldn't be there all day; my son came daily and had lunch with me, then spent a couple of hours with me; my daughter-in-law arrived around 9 PM every night, after she got the three boys to bed, and would stay with me until 11 or 11:30 PM. She even had the pleasure of being with me the night I had a severe reaction to a new anti-nausea medication, and I thank God she was there! My gynecologist was a Godsend, coming by every day, some days visiting twice, and giving me encouragement and support, always going above and beyond what was expected of any doctor. I looked forward to seeing him because I knew he was in my corner and would do whatever he could to help me beat this.

At some point during what was turning out to be a long and drawn-out hospital stay, my gynecologist came in to give me the best news ever. All of my biopsies, slides, washers and the PET showed that the cancer was contained within the cervix and that they had removed all of it during the surgery. I almost shook with relief. It has not spread! I am clean everywhere else! I am so blessed! After seven days of complications and severe nausea, on August 14th I was finally going home. Unfortunately, I had to leave with my drainage tube (it was removed four days later), but my spirits could not be dampened. I was accompanied by the greatest news I could have hoped for.

And the blessings from my loved ones continued with homemade dinners from my boss's wife and several friends, visits and phone calls and text messages. It was those small, simple gestures that helped me get through that first week.

During my weekly follow-up appointments with my gynecologist, I decided that, considering I had not had a good experience with the senior oncologist I had seen, I should pursue getting a second opinion from another oncologist at a major Chicago hospital. When the day of my second opinion arrived, I was extremely anxious. What would he say? What if he had a difference of opinion? What would I do then?

It was an hour-and-a-half drive and, arriving an hour early, the reality set in again. I could see a room off to the side with a stack of masks and shelves of wigs on display.

Germ masks and wigs. I had cancer and I couldn't escape that fact. There were pamphlets all around about cancer and how to tell children that you have cancer and how to tell children when someone they love dies of cancer. All I could do was think of my three grandsons and I started crying. I pulled myself together, checked in and I was escorted inside right away. Even better, everyone was so nice. A very different experience than those three visits I'd had with the other oncologist.

I first met with the nurse, then the resident and finally the specialist. He asked me several standard questions, questions that I was getting used to answering, as they seemed to be asked every time. Then came his opinion. He said that, with this type of cancer and how quickly it spreads, chemo was a definite. He also felt that pelvic and brain radiation were not justified at this point, but he cautioned me that he needed to review the slides and pictures of the PET scan and would call me the following afternoon. I left with positive feelings that it appeared I only had chemo left to get through before I would be at the end of this particular path in my life's journey, the path known as cancer.

The next day, as he said he would, the oncologist from that major hospital called and, again, my world took a few steps backward. He said he had met with another oncologist and a radiation gynecologist about my case. First, they all agreed that chemo must be done (both Cisplatin and Etoposide). But then he said that they all agreed I should have a head MRI, as they believe the PET scan does not always pick up the cancer in the brain area, especially with small cell cancers. He said this should be done prior to treatment, as the results could change my treatment plan.

He continued that, after having discussed the pros and cons of brain radiation, he felt this should be considered at the end of my treatment. Studies have shown a 5% improvement, but again, this is based off small cell lung cancer. Lastly, the doctors he talked to urged that pelvic radiation should also be considered, although there are mixed feelings on this controversial, preventative treatment, and there are no good studies on its effectiveness. We discussed an overview of what his treatment plan would be. He also said he felt, because he did not do the surgery on me himself, it was difficult for him to know how completely everything was performed. But because I was young and healthy, he wanted to pursue aggressive treatment. This, he said, was to give me my best chance of survival. "Survival" I have come to have a love/hate relationship with that word!

I hung up the phone and, just like that, my positive outlook flew right out the window. It had only been three weeks since I had wonderfully, mercifully been told that my cancer had not spread and now I just had a doctor tell me I needed an MRI to rule out brain cancer. I thought I was past this part and now I was thinking this was a relentless disease that will never be gone. My head had always known the challenges and the stresses and the frustrations that were in store for me with this disease, but my heart had been fighting valiantly to stay positive. Worrying about this second opinion had frayed my nerves and I was still trying to heal from my surgery, four weeks before. I was debating whether to get a port, deciding what oncologist I should trust with my life, investigating the process of getting a wig. Every single one of these things, just 6-7 short weeks ago, I'd never imagined I'd be doing. It was too much. I was tired and frustrated and beaten down and emotionally drowning.

On September 6, my gynecologist, along with the original oncology group I had seen, presented my case to the Tumor Board. It took four days before we were finally able to talk. He told me that the board also recommended chemo with the same two chemo drugs and that they were reluctant to pursue any type of pelvic or brain radiation at this point. Their plan was to start chemo as soon as possible, then repeat the PET scan and reassess whether additional chemo or radiation would be needed. They did, however, agree that I must have a brain MRI as soon as possible, before starting any treatment plan.

I was lucky enough to get an appointment on September 12th at 8:00 AM, and I was delighted there was no prep involved. I could even get over my dislike of being in that tube for more than 30 minutes, without being able to move, knowing that I didn't have to do the prep that made me so sick. When I arrived they took me in and, once again, I had a great tech who explained the process and assured me he would keep talking me through it. I laid down on the gurney, they placed my head in this plastic cage and we did a few trial runs, then we were off. He would come on and tell me, "Ok, this one will be for four minutes." I would then start counting in my head. Done. He would then come on and say again, "This one will be for four minutes," and so on until I was finished. My sister and brother-in-law had met my significant other and me at the hospital for every test I had had through this ordeal and this time was no different. Knowing it was going to be two days before I heard any results, I enjoyed breakfast with them and, yes, a great cup of coffee.

Shortly after getting home, my cell rang and I could see it was my gynecologist calling. My heart began beating incredibly quickly as I answered. It was his nurse. I said, "Please tell me you are not calling me with bad news." She told me that my doctor had come flying out of his office and told her to call me right away, that he had the results of my MRI and they were NORMAL. NO SIGNS of cancer! She said she had never seen him move so fast. I had received this blessed news only three short hours after my test and I excitedly began telling my family and friends.

On September 14th, I was cleared for chemo. Now the final part of, at least what I hope to be, only one chapter of my life begins. I have recently decided, after much discussion with my gynecologist, to see an oncologist closer to where I live. With that said, the whole process starts again. My medical records need to be sent, I'll hope he can get me in right away and I'll be praying that he has the same vision as the others. Above all, I hope he is a compassionate doctor and that the center where I'll be receiving my chemo is one of kindness and consideration for me and for all of those who have had to take this detour in their life's journey. My chemo should begin in the next few weeks and I especially pray that I haven't waited too long. As my gynecologist explained in such an easy-to-understand way: there are hundreds of terrorists in the subway (the terrorists being the tumor), the officials (doctors) come in and kill them all and, as they retreat, there's still the question of whether there could possibly be one more terrorist that wasn't killed, out there somewhere, hiding. Simply, I need the chemo to be sure all the cancer cells have been found and killed!

There are a lot of unknowns in my life now, including my final treatment plan, but I do know one thing for sure. My life has changed forever. I used to always tell people, "Until you have a child, you will never experience the love you will feel when it is your own child or grandchild." The same holds true for this disease. Until you have been given those three words, "YOU HAVE CANCER," you can't possibly understand the true impact of what those words mean.

I think back to the night my daughter-in-law and I sat down with my two oldest grandchildren, Tyler, who is 11, and Jacob, who is 7, to explain to them what I have and what to expect. During the conversation, Tyler asked if my cancer was the "dying kind." Fighting to not cry, we took deep breaths and said we hoped not and that we would do everything we could to make sure I will be ok. When I was leaving, Tyler went to hug me and it was a little bit of a light hug. He turned to me and asked, "Is it contagious?" "Oh sweetie, no, it is not," I said. And then he gave me the biggest hug! I truly live for those three wonderful, spirited boys and I am positive that this is what will get me through all of this. I want to be at every baseball game, every basketball game, every prom night, all of their weddings and at the births of their own children; every milestone they go through. My family and friends and my significant other will be an amazing support system as I walk this road, but my son and my three grandsons have taken my heart to heights beyond imagination. The mere thought of not being here for them is simply not an option.

As I begin, what I hope to be, my final walk in this journey of healing and becoming cancer free, I truly feel blessed for my family and friends. My significant other has been by my side, taken me to every appointment and has gone above and beyond to take care of me and support me. My family is there consistently, either stopping by or calling daily, and my brother and sister have been rocks for me. They have come through for me over and over. My friends, so many of them, are either calling or picking me up to get me out of the house on what I call, "field trips," or they are making us meals and dropping them off. I am not sure when my one friend started this but, to keep my spirits up, she began texting me a nightly "knock knock" joke and a "how was your day?" text that continues to this day. I can't explain what those text messages and her constant support have meant. I would be lost without my daughter-in-law and I am so blessed to have her in my life and as the mother of my grandchildren. My son always tries to be so strong. If I could go back in time to when I was raising him as a single mother, I probably would have changed a lot of things. But I hope he knows I did the best that I could and always tried to make life better for him. I love him more than words could describe.

I am truly blessed to have my boss as a friend. He has been supportive, proactive and with me every step of the way. He surprised me with specially made t-shirts for our employees and me, to show support, which they continue to wear to this day. He has lifted so much stress off my shoulders throughout this journey and couldn't have done this without him. He told me that he would go through this with me. If I lose my hair, he would shave his off, and knowing him, he would! My significant other has been by my side, taken me to every appointment and has gone above and beyond to take care of me and support me.

When I started writing this story, I had not started my treatment and have since just completed chemo. My treatment began October 3rd for 3 days in a row, 5-6 hours each day, then 18 days off and so on for 4 rounds, ending *my last day of chemo on December 7, 2012. At this point, unless they strongly recommend radiation, I have declined. I remember my first day of chemo. I cried all the way there and almost the entire 6-7 hours I was there that day. I struggled with each round, but the worst was that first round. My significant other thought I was going to die, and during that first 2 weeks, I truly wanted to. I thought about suicide, ever so briefly. That is truly when God blessed me again and gave me the strength to get through those dark days. I will have my post chemo PET scan in February of 2013, and pray it will be clear, as well as my next brain MRI, due in a few weeks.*

People often ask me, "Do you mind if I tell so-and-so?" I do not care if others spread the word about my illness. I feel that the more people who know, the better because, if they care about me, they will say some prayers for me and you can never have too many of those! Besides this, though, it also brings awareness to this rare cancer on which there is no data, no protocol and no research because we are only 1 in a 1,000, and very, very special!

The cards and messages continued to come weekly for 5 months straight. I can't put into words what they meant to me. My good friend continued her "nightly knock, knock jokes" through my last round of chemo and we finally stopped at 150 jokes. It's a good thing otherwise she was going to have to buy a joke book. You truly find out who your true friends are and how many people you touch through life that care enough to reach out.

I truly believe that, at this point, I have so many people praying for me that God is up there, throwing his hands up in the air and saying, "Enough already, I get it, you want me to leave her down there for another twenty to thirty years! Ok, fine! I hear you! Consider it done!"

I BeLIeVE!!!!!

A special addendum as of April 13, 2013: I still beLIeVE, BUT when pain took me to the hospital, multiple recurrences were found. My cancer is back and I wonder, really, if it was ever gone in February, when I received my great news that I was "clear." I now have 3 spots on my pancreas, 1 spot in my pelvis and one spot on my brain. Chemo started again on April 26th for, most likely, 6 rounds and we will repeat all Scans/MRI after the 3rd round to determine the next step. Although this is devastating news, I still beLIeVE that God has a plan for me to stay right here and allow me to have the miracle I pray for so much. I BeLIeVE...now in MIRACLES too!!

Michelle Peeple's Story:

August 3, 2012. The day that I heard the words, "You have cancer." Not just any kind of cancer, "You have a rare cancer that, in my thirty years of practice, I have never seen or diagnosed." I was told I needed to see an oncologist immediately. I began a Google search of Small Cell Neuroendocrine Carcinoma of the Cervix. At that very moment, any thought I had that this was going to be solved easily was shattered. I basically went into shock reading the words "rare," "aggressive," "chemotherapy," "radiation," "lack of research." The words went on and on and my mind raced on and on. I found a link on a cervical cancer website that was written about Jennifer Dunmoyer. It was the first article I had found that gave me HOPE!

I met with my oncologist who sent me for a PET scan, MRI, and then port placement surgery so I could begin chemotherapy. All of these events happened within a week. It was like my world was spinning out of control. I just went through the motions of life, not living, just existing. I believed in God. I always trusted Him and I knew to turn to Him. But instead of letting Him be in control, I tried to control my emotions and my feelings to a point that I pushed God away from the situation and the hurt I was feeling. I did this, not only to God, but to everyone. I smiled and said I was fine, but inside my heart was broken and I was aware that my life, as I knew it, wasn't ever going to be the same.

More Google searching led to more depression and hopelessness. I turned to Facebook to look for a page dedicated to this type of cancer. I was thrilled to find that one existed! From that moment I began "meeting" women from all over the world who had this rare form of cervical cancer. I felt an immediate assurance that I would be cared for and supported by other women who knew exactly what I would be going through during treatment. These women could answer questions for me, refer me to women in the group who'd had similar experiences and, most of all, support and love me through my treatment.

My tumor was around 6-7 cm and I was staged at 1b2. My treatment plan was to shrink the tumor and then have surgery followed by radiation. I received 6 rounds of chemo in Amarillo, Texas at Harrington Cancer Center. Each round was a 3-day regimen of Cisplatin and Etoposide. I had each 3-day round 3 weeks apart. I began to have hearing loss, which caused the doctor to switch my chemo cocktail to Carboplatin and Etoposide for the last two treatment rounds.

My soul and my relationship with God became stronger than ever. I had many hours of heart to heart talks with my Savior. I could go on and on about this transformation in my life. I gave myself the title of "WARRIOR." I even dressed up as a WARRIOR with my mohawk and had my daughter, who was studying photography, take a picture of me that way. I started to blog my experiences. http://motleypeeples.blogspot.com. I hope that they will inspire and help others going through this battle.

Exodus 14:14

The LORD will fight for you; you need only to be still.

On January 16, 2013, I went in to have a robotic radical hysterectomy. The surgery, that was supposed to take a few hours, ended up taking 9 1/2 hours and leaving me with a slice down my abdomen from below my chest to my pelvis. I also received 8 units of blood during that time. I woke up in ICU that evening with a lot of pain and confusion. I remained in the hospital for over a week, due to complications. I finally went home only to return again a few days later with more complications. I spent most of the month of January and first week of February in room 318. I ended up in the same room every time I returned. My pathology report from my surgery showed 45 lymph nodes removed, no evidence of disease, no malignancy and clear margins. Cervix tumor had extensive vascular invasion at the base of the tumor, but it was contained with no malignancy. In other words, no surrounding tissue had disease. I felt sure that I had fought and won. My doctor then suggested radiation treatment. I'd had so many internal problems that going in this direction was not what I wanted to do. I was still healing after over a month.

I decided it was time to visit Dr. Michael Frumovitz at MD Anderson. I had visited with him a few times during treatment and he was always interested and helpful. He was the mentor to the Sorority of Hope, and actively worked to conduct meaningful research for this rare disease. I went to visit him in March of 2013.

Dr. Frumovitz performed a biopsy at that visit. The results came back that it I, once again, had Small Cell Neuroendocrine Carcinoma. Without getting into too many details, my disease has spread throughout my body. Nodules were found in various places, including my lungs. Dr F. now has me on a different chemo regimen, Taxotere and Avastin, every 3 weeks. I have done 3 rounds of this combination and seem to be responding with success in my clinical appointments in Amarillo. I am going back to Houston for another PET/CT scan in June. I know I have more chemotherapy in my future and radiation is still another possibility. I know that my future will always have this disease as a part of its reality.

I plan on continuing my "incurable" optimism. I have a very supportive family, a loving husband and two teenaged daughters who have also had to live with this disease and how it is affecting me. My community has been very supportive and caring as well. To give back to those in my *small town of Dalhart, Texas, my husband and I started a fund to help people in our community who travel for cancer treatments. We live over 80 miles from the cancer centers in Amarillo and it's 684 miles from Dalhart to Houston. Our fund is called the Twilight Fund. Yes, I am a Twilight saga fan! We are on Facebook;*

https://www.facebook.com/TwilightFund

Chapter 7

We are all familiar with the phrase, "6 degrees of separation," or today, they say it is more like 3 degrees, thanks to Social Media. That couldn't be truer than it is with our group. It's one of the most amazing aspects of what we, as a whole, and the tenacity of a few, have been able to accomplish.

In the beginning of this journey, it was very apparent to Melanie and me that this disease could very likely come back to either both or at least one of us. 50/50 odds. So early on, with the direction of a newly found Cancer Comrade who was losing her battle and looking for anything that might help, the women were introduced to MD Anderson in Texas. We were given the name of a Dr. M. Frumovitz and the name, email and phone number of a woman by the name of Carla Moore, who was the key point of contact for the MD Anderson Small Cell Cervical Cancer Trial, headed by Dr. Frumovitz. We passed this information on to any new sister, as well as the ones we already had, hoping to get those in need of treatment into the trial, or at least get some expert help in this area. As far as we could tell, these people were the closest thing to SCCC "specialists" we would find. These were definitely the only people with a trial for SCCC of any kind. This was January 14th, 2009. As the group grew, the information was passed on from person to person, until we eventually found out the trial had to be dropped. Because of the rarity of SCCC, there were never enough subjects in the same geographical area, with the same stage of treatment, to have a successful trial. It was too expensive for the patients to relocate so they could be monitored by MD Anderson. That was very disheartening to find out. But it wasn't going to stop this group from hoping or stop one particular supporter from pushing. Without ever knowing about the group's link to MDA, this supporter did her own research and legwork with the biggest motivation one could have; She needed to save her sister.

Jessica McGinnis's story:

"What do you mean you won't take my money?"

"I'm sorry ma'am, but there is no research being done for Small Cell Cervical Cancer. We don't even have any information about it, so your money wouldn't go towards that particular cancer. Have you tried the National Cervical Cancer Coalition?"

"Yes, I already tried. No luck there either. Thanks anyway."

After calling and emailing numerous organizations for the goal of finding information or to contribute money to the research of SCCC, I realized I couldn't find anything because nothing was being done. There was no information. No good information. No positive information. No hope. Nothing for me to bring back to my sister to help ease her fears. This was July 2010.

I kept searching. I Googled and read and Googled and read some more. I kept coming upon MD Anderson, ranked #1 cancer center. I figured if anyone could help me, they could. I reviewed the bios of a few of the gynecologists and choose Dr. Pedro Ramirez. It was a shot in the dark, but I figured it was worth a shot. Dr. Ramirez referred me to the development office and a representative emailed me. MJ Suehs just happened to be coming to Philly in October and would LOVE to meet my sister, Jen, and me to discuss our philanthropic interests! Boy, oh, boy was I excited! Nervous as heck, but excited!

I really only had about $50 to donate. Who would fly across the county for a $50 donation?? Oh no! I'll bet she thinks I'm rich and want to donate thousands!! Jen and I just decided to go along with whatever was happening and see where it took us.

Upon meeting with MJ, she said she would see what they could do. She started speaking to Dr. Michael Frumovitz, who offered to help spearhead the efforts. In his professional opinion, an online, global registry for physicians, as well as patients, would be the best "bang for our buck." With so few patients available, traditional clinical trials just wouldn't work. This was it. This was our shot. Someone was not only willing to listen, but willing to help! Fundraising began immediately to help fill our fund! Custom, silicon SCCC bracelets with the words, "Rare But There, Help for Hope, Hope for Help" were made to help facilitate funds. After this, the SCCC sisterhood took off with ideas of t-shirts, magnets, walks, benefits, etc. The money started coming in from around the world.

While SCCC is rare, these women are there. To the few it affects, it becomes everything. It becomes their life, and they will never be the same. All they want is the opportunity to be alive and well, and heard and helped like the more common, widely publicized cancers. They want hope too. They are now getting it! Newly diagnosed sisters now have hope! They do not have to feel alone. They can know that SOMEONE is doing SOMETHING to help. Thank you to MD Anderson for opening your hearts to help and for all of our family and friends for opening your wallets. Thank you for your prayers and your love.

While most people say that hard work, perseverance and a positive attitude will get you far, I say, God will get you farther. I thank God for allowing all of this to happen and guiding our steps along the way. I thank God for saving Jen's life. She has just celebrated her 2-year cancer-free anniversary!! We have raised over $130,000 and the funds continue to come in. God is in control and has allowed all of this to happen, for his purposes.

Proverbs 3:6: "In all thy ways, acknowledge him, and he shall direct thy paths." Thank you, God, for directing me to MD Anderson.

In 2012, as was mentioned in a few stories prior, an amazing thing happened. More than 40 sisters and supporters came together to meet in person in Las Vegas, some for the very first time. As an outsider watching this group, you would probably never have known that most were meeting in person for the very first time at this gathering. It was as if the group of women had always known each other. There had been the first meeting in New York City in 2011 that had sparked this annual event. But something magical happened that weekend in Vegas, for many attending in 2012. Bonds were forged and special friendships begun. There something magical in the air that you could almost touch. Maybe it was hope? Possibly faith? Definitely strength. But, you could feel it. At a very special dinner, while in Vegas, Dr. Michael Frumovitz came walking through the door and into our lives. He came to meet us and share the news of the upcoming events concerning our research fund. Here is his take on that night, the research and the group.

In Dr. M Frumovitz's Words:

As I sat in a private dining room in Las Vegas, surrounded by 19 women with small and large cell cervical cancer (easily the largest gathering in history of women with this rare disease), I took a moment to reflect upon how I ended up there. Nine months earlier, I had been working in my office in Houston one afternoon, when a woman from the development office called me.

"I have a group of women who want to raise money for research in small and large cell cancer of the cervix," she said. "Are you interested in accepting it?"

An opening like that would obviously interest any researcher. In addition to research funds materializing from seemingly nowhere, I had reason to be attracted in such a directed gift, having years earlier been the principal investigator on the only attempt to perform a clinical trial for women with small cell cervical cancer. Unfortunately, owing to the rarity of this disease, that study failed to enroll more than 3 patients in 2 years and the sponsoring pharmaceutical company was forced to close it. So I had some interest in the disease. Plus, free money for research. "Let's talk," I replied.

We met the next day and she outlined the donors' vision for the funds. "Translational research aimed at finding a cure for small and large cell neuroendocrine cancer of the cervix," I was told. Translational research is a bit of a catchall term for any basic science or animal research that is focused on discoveries that quickly can be moved from the laboratory to clinical care. Some refer to this type of research as "bench to bedside," as the laboratory setting is sometimes referred to as "bench research."

I assumed it was a very large donation. We both knew to perform good laboratory research we would need $500,000 to start. Just to start. I would learn that a couple of women with this disease and their supporters and families had found one another on Facebook. Energized by their numbers, albeit small numbers, they were going to raise the money via small donations, bake sales, sponsored walks, and the like. They thought, in a few years, they could raise $50,000. Maybe $75,000 if things went their way. A "nickel and dime" approach to fundraising, if you will. Certainly, I do not mean to imply that $50,000 or $75,000 is negligible. Those are obviously substantial sums of money. Sadly, for translational research, that type of funding won't last three months.

"I'm not sure what we can do with that type of money."

Other than a cure for this terrible disease, what was really lacking in the field of Neuroendocrine Cervical Cancers? In the end we decided there was a paucity of basic information. Information that could help both women with this disease to learn about their diagnosis as well as help researchers trying to get a handle on this disease. For what we thought was going to be a limited budget, we landed on a website as the best means to achieve both goals. The website would, first and foremost, serve as an educational venue for women with small and large cell cervical cancers, as very little credible information exists on the Internet. When a scared woman turns to Google to look for information on this rare disease, she is left longing. The website would become the main online source of information on small and large cell cervical cancers for women trying to figure out exactly what was going on with their bodies. We could help newly diagnosed women find facts about the disease, find women who could help support them, and empower them with information about this cancer.

Once the website was up and running, we would use its visibility as the only place on the Internet to find information on this disease and parlay that into research by advertising our patient registry. The registry would recruit women with this disease and their doctors to send us all of their information, from diagnosis through treatment. If we could compile information in treatment successes and failures among a large group of women with this disease, we could then begin to detect trends in treatments that worked and those that did not work. We would then focus on steering women to those therapies that offer the best chance of survival. We pitched this idea to the potential donors and were met with gratitude for taking up the cause.

Which takes me back to my night in Las Vegas. The women blasted by that $75,000 goal in a less than a year. In less than nine months, actually. With such incredible efforts to raise money so quickly, I felt obliged to fly out to Vegas to meet them and let them know what we were planning for their hard work. I thought I would walk into the dining room, give my pep talk, grab a quick bite, and then leave. What ensued, however, was one of the most gratifying experiences in my eleven years in gynecologic oncology.

I entered a room filled with some of the most incredible women I have ever had the honor of meeting. These women had built a bond using social media and now were face-to-face with one another. The outpouring of love and support that had been merely virtual in the months before, was now real and palpable. I sat in my chair, awestruck, as I watched survivors supporting newly diagnosed. I watched women currently being treated seeking advice and guidance from those who had been through the same. There were women in the room, who we knew were likely on their last vacation, being treated as fellow cancer survivors for the first time probably since they were diagnosed. When you have a rare disease, and have been told you're 1 in a million (and not in a lucky way), being surrounded by 19 other 1 in a millions like yourself must have been a most exhilarating experience. Reassuring. Comforting. Liberating. And I consider myself privileged to have been part of their experience and to have shared in that outpouring of love and support.

And now, six months after Vegas, we are at almost $250,000 raised. We can now actually start thinking about funding some of that expensive translational research. We can start thinking about zeroing in on therapeutics that may work for women with this disease. We can start dreaming of clinical trials and cures for women with small and large cell cervical cancers. What happens in Vegas stays in Vegas? I'm not so sure.

Our group has grown in leaps and bounds, so has our research fund. You may have noticed that when others have mentioned the research fund, the totals have varied. This is because the fund grows daily. Well-wishers and supporters give generously all the time and the members of our group work tirelessly to come up with ways to raise any amount they can. As stated earlier, "Together We Are a Movement." This group, although relatively small in numbers, is overflowing with sheer determination. As this book goes to print, we have just come home from our 2013 annual gathering in Las Vegas. At dinner, Dr. F. and his teammate, Dr. Burzawa, told us that the tumor registry had been approved that very day. We currently have a website, for informational purposes, that was donated by a friend of one of the sisters. The registry link will be posted on this site and all of the funds raised can now go to maintaining our registry and research, which is on the horizon. We were told of a possible nationwide trial we might be eligible for as well. Great things are happening. You can be more than certain of this...we will never give up! With the help of MD Anderson, Dr. Frumovitz and Dr. Burzawa, we will accomplish our goal of finding treatment protocols and, maybe someday, a cure. One thing is positive, Dr. Frumovitz is our guardian angel and we will forever be grateful to him and his team's work. Thank you for believing in us. Whether it is 6 degrees or 3, together we are connected, and no one is alone.

Chapter 8

Along this path we have lost some of our "comrades." Those we have lost and the words they have left for us show that our journeys are much the same, though the endings may be different. As they did in their lives, they have given us inspiration and hope to continue this battle and honor them by doing so. We remember our fallen sisters by sharing some of their stories and spreading the hope they wished to share.

Veronica Doyle O'Meara

Hi sisters :-) My name is Veronica, I'm 32 and I'm from Tipperary in Ireland. I was diagnosed with SCCC in Oct 2009. It had spread to lymph nodes in my pelvis and groin. I started my treatment at St. Luke's Hospital in Dublin. I started with 3 rounds of chemo every 3 weeks, Cisplatin and Etoposide. I had an MRI after 2 rounds and the tumor had shrunk from 10 cm to 6 cm, so that was good news. I went through Hell with the chemo. I had it for 5 days every 3 weeks and that was a very tough. I then started the radiotherapy in Jan 09. I had 28 external to pelvis. After that the plan was to do 3 internal radiation treatments. So I went down to theatre, had my spinal and was sedated, came round about 20 minutes later only to have the doctor tell me that they couldn't do it because the tumor was still too big. It was covering the opening of my cervix. I had 3 more external radiation treatments after that. Then that was it. My oncologist discharged me from St. Luke's and said there was no more that they could do. He contacted my surgeon at Waterford Regional Hospital to discuss a hysterectomy, so I said, "Fine, that's ok. I can do that." Only to find out that the only surgery that I could have was a total pelvic clear out and leave me with a urostomy bag and a colostomy bag. I told them no. There was not a hope would I have it. The surgeon wasn't even in favor of it, he said there is even a high mortality rate with it, and he said even if I did have it, I'd spend 6 months recovering and then the cancer could show up somewhere else, and that would have been a waste of 6 months, as he put it. So he basically just told me to enjoy what life you have left. But the way I look at it is, that's just one man and his opinion. God brought me into the world and God knows when I'll be leaving, not a surgeon :-) So that's my story in a nutshell. I'm not angry with anyone, I'm happier in my life now than I've ever been and I have SCCC. Yes, some of you might find that hard to understand, but that's just how I feel. I have found Jesus again and I know he is now carrying my cross for me. I know it is God that has filled me with this peace. I believe that Jesus is the Divine Healer and I believe that He will heal me if it is His Holy will. So, I'm off to Lourdes in the morning and I will keep you all in my prayers at all times. I forgot to mention above that I had a PET scan about 6 weeks ago and my lymph nodes were clear, so the radiation did work on those. I still have a 3 cm tumor on my cervix, but the cancer hasn't spread. I know I'm very lucky and blessed to be able to sit here today and write this, and I thank you, God, for that. Love to you all. xxxxx

Michelle Planten

Hi Sisters. I was diagnosed in October 2009, after a routine PAP smear led to a biopsy because my gynecologist didn't like the looks of the lesions on my cervix. I think he knew it was cancer, but he knew what an anxious psycho I can be. lol. The biopsy was done on Wednesday, September 30th, and my gynecologist came knocking on my front door on October 5th to give me the news. Yes, he came to my house. Isn't that saying, "You are dying"? I almost passed out from crying. I did not understand just how bad my diagnosis was until I went on the Internet to find out more about this cancer. Even my doctor didn't tell me how rare and aggressive this type is. I cried every day for I don't even know how long. Every time I looked at my kids, I just started crying.

I have 3 kids and a wonderful husband. My oldest is 22 and he is in the Army, stationed in Hawaii, and being deployed in July. Then I started over with my current husband, and we have a 7 year-old son named Julian, who happens to be autistic. Then my youngest is 4 year-old, Myah. She has an amazing birth story in itself, but that is for another post, I guess. lol.

My treatments began with a radical hysterectomy. Since I didn't actually have a tumor, but lesions instead, they could do surgery right away, which they did on October 16th. What Hell it was recovering from that! Then I started chemo and radiation on November 30th. I had Cisplatin and Etoposide. I went through Hell with that as well. Nothing, and I mean nothing, has been easy with any of these treatments. I finished that treatment on February 8th, and I was so happy it was all over! Then I was sent for a CT scan on my abdomen because I told the doctor I was having pains in my stomach area. I thought I was constipated, and he sent me for a CT scan! My abdominal area was clear, but they caught a look at the bottom of my right lung on that scan, and there was a 4 mm spot. So, I was sent for a CT scan of my lungs, and one more 4 mm spot was found. They said they were too small to diagnose, so nothing to do. However, they did find 2 other spots on my lumbar spine, and one on my scapula (wing bone). My gynecological oncologist told me to find another doctor because he really didn't know what to do. GREAT, thanks Doc.

I've found a wonderful medical oncologist now. She has put me on the 2nd line treatment for this cancer when it is in the lungs, which is a chemo called Topotecan. I pray and cry every day that this works. I have only had one round so far. My new doctor said this one wouldn't make me sick like the Cisplatin did. YEAH RIGHT! I was sick as a dog. So they had to give me all kinds of pre-meds just like the first time, and also anti-nausea drugs to take home.

I don't know if this will work or not. I hope it does. If it doesn't, she said she has something else in mind. What scares me is that this cancer was caught early in the beginning and spread while I was on chemo, so I am scared to death that I have a supersonic strain that will not respond to treatments and just kill me.

I don't know how I would have done without the women I met on Cancer Comrades. They are with me either by listening or sharing their hopes or trying to teach me faith. I am still scared every day that I will die from this cancer. I hope one day to not be scared anymore.

Sharon Thompson

Hello Ladies, I am 38 years old, from UK with 2 children, aged 19 and 17. I was diagnosed with SCCC in September 2008. I hadn't had a smear/PAP test since the year 2000. I *had a large tumor diagnosed stage 4B after a biopsy was done, which showed small cell and squamous cell cancer, so a bit unusual. I also had a lymph node in my neck, which was about 5cm². Treatment was started within a few weeks, 3 weekly rounds of Etoposide and Carboplatin chemotherapy, for 3 cycles (18 weeks) then I had a CT scan which showed that the tumors had not shrunk. I then started the following 3 weeks afterwards CAV chemo infusions and injections, 3 cycles again (18 weeks). Another CT scan revealed that the tumors were still growing and a new one had developed in the right ovary. I then had external radiotherapy 5 days a week for 5 weeks on my abdomen and 5 days a week for 4 weeks on my neck area. I then had another CT scan, which showed not a lot had happened. At this time, my oncologist referred me to the Royal Marsden Cancer Hospital in Sutton Surrey, UK for Phase 1 drug trials.*

Participating in Phase 1 drug trials is a laborious task, mostly because this is the first time the drugs have been used in humans. I attended lots of appointments before I was actually given the drugs. There were consent forms, marker CT and MRI scans, MUGA heart scans, etc. The hospital was 90 miles away from my house.

I eventually got started on a drug called Cediranib. It is a drug designed to stop blood flow to tumors, thus making them not grow anymore. I got on very well on this drug for a couple of months until, in December 2009, I went into the hospital in pain and had constipation. The CT scan showed that the blood flow had been stopped to part of my bowel, so the drug was stopped immediately and I received strong intravenous antibiotics to clear the problem, which, luckily, it did. I was sent home and a month later attended the

Marsden for more of the appointments, marker scans, etc, and then was put on another trial drug called JNJ25390. This new drug was designed to alter the DNA of cancer cells. I must admit I didn't feel well whilst on this drug. Also, the vaginal bleeding and discharge reappeared and I began to get pain. After a month of being on JNJ I had a CT scan which revealed that the tumor in my cervix had grown and another had appeared in my other ovary, and these 3 were showing as one big mass. Also a new tumor appeared on the tail of my pancreas and one on the side of my face, which was a lymph node 1cm². The drug was stopped immediately.

In the weeks after this appointment I was admitted into a surgical ward at my local hospital with pain and constipation. My GP had thought I had a blockage in my bowel, although it turned out that it was probably the tumor in the pancreas stopping my large intestine from working properly. They did a CT scan, which showed all the tumors in my abdomen had grown even bigger and the doctors actually said, "Sharon you look a lot better on the outside than you do on the inside!" I saw a palliative care nurse to discuss pain relief. I am now taking morphine, 20 mg slow release, twice a day and regularly take laxatives to help my bowel. I also went into the local gynecological hospital the week after this visit due to a large vaginal bleed. At this point these new doctors did consider surgery but changed their minds due to the risks. Risks to them or me? I was given tranexamic acid to stop the bleeding. It works a bit but I'm always bleeding still, which is rather annoying.

I again went back to the Marsden when I was better to see if they would consider me for another drug trial. The professor I saw said that another drug trial would probably cause more harm than good, so he referred me back to my local hospital for palliative chemotherapy called Taxol, given in weekly infusions.

I started this new Taxol 4 weeks ago and, I must admit, I am feeling fine on it. I have already noticed that the tumor on my face has gotten much smaller and I can hardly see it or feel it now, which I can only assume is good news. I have 3 more weekly chemo sessions planned then I assume I will be scanned to see if there are any changes.

I am still taking the slow release morphine and the tranexamic acid twice daily. I am pain-free mostly. I have had a few problems with night sweats, but it could be the weather. My bowel appears to be working OK and I no longer take the laxatives. I have also improved my diet. I am not feeling ill at all. I feel fantastic. I have been carrying on living my life to the fullest. I think my hair has gotten thin, but I'm not bothered about that so long as the tumors are shrinking. My partner did say to me yesterday my tummy looks a lot flatter, so here's to hoping!

I think I have defied the odds of still being here. I was given 6 months to live in April 2009. Anyone who knows me knows what a positive person I am, and I intend to carry on being like I am. This disease is a mystery to all the oncologists I have met. I am aware that in UK they don't like to do surgery unless they absolutely have to. Perhaps that's why I am still here. Who knows? And maybe one day we will know.

Rosie Fiercefighter Lindberg-Lakso

Hi Ladies,

I am so thankful to be a part of your group. You have literally been a lifesaver, true angel ladies!!!! I was invited to the group, although I actually was diagnosed with Large Cell Neuroendocrine Carcinoma of the Cervix, which is even more rare than small cell. I still have not been able to connect with anyone with my same diagnosis. I am planning on starting my own Facebook group in hopes of finding someone out there.

I am a mother of two, Prince who is 3 years old and Isis who is 23 months. They are only 14 months apart and truly my little angels. We were not quite financially equipped to have both so close together, but if I didn't have them when I did they would not be here! I truly believe everything happens for a reason. I have been with their father, William, for 11 years. We are not officially married, but unofficially we are! He is the love of my life, he drives me crazy sometimes, but I love him soooooo much. I also have a wonderful job as an Interpretive Guide at the Minnesota Zoo.

I was diagnosed with HPV 10 years ago, with just mild dysplasia, and had normal PAPs all the way up to this past February 23rd, 2010. I had a very abnormal pap and needed a colposcopy, which was scheduled for March 15th. On March 17th, I got the call that it was cancer and I needed to see the OB/GYN oncologist, Dr. Argenta, on April 5th. On April 8th, my PET scan revealed it was only on my cervix, THANK GOD!!!! On April 13th, I had a radical Da Vinci hysterectomy. They took everything but my ovaries. AND NO LYMPH NODE INVOLVEMENT!!! Surgery went better than expected! I thought I was in the clear. On April 19th I found out I was not so lucky. The good news was, Dr. Argenta felt he removed all the cancer, the bad news was *the cancer I "had," was Large Cell Carcinoma of the Cervix. So rare, he had never worked with anyone with this type of cancer, and I was now labeled a "special case."*

We were all terrified. Everything I read about Large Cell was devastating, and I couldn't find anyone else around who had this cancer or anyone who knew how to treat it. It was hard at first, but I was drawn by the fact that I was currently CANCER FREE, and determined to stay that way! So I truly believe in the power of the mind over body. I am in control of this cancer it is not in control of me! So I trusted to stay with my doctor team because they were consulting MD Anderson in Texas for treatment options.

So on May 24th I started a chemo (Cisplatin) and radiation combo for six weeks. I got my chemo on Mondays and radiation Monday through Friday. Surprisingly, it really wasn't that bad. I got a little diarrhea, but my body handled it amazingly well. My follow-up with Dr. Argenta went well. He said my body was healing well from the radiation.

I got a break in July to enjoy my kids, work and enjoy summer a little bit. Then, on August 3rd, I had another PET scan that again revealed that I was and am still CANCER FREE! But then the fight began again. I started heavy doses of chemo, Cisplatin and Etoposide, on August 10th. Wow, big difference!! This is a lot harder on my body. I have lost my hair and I have become anemic, but still my doctors are amazed at how well my body is handling the treatment. I only have one more round left on the week of Oct. 11th. God willing, this will be my last treatment ever!

Beyond my treatment I will be starting my healing journey. I am going to take my health more seriously and take time for just me. Join me in the search for alternative cancer therapies and healing therapies. I am not a hippie, but I do believe that there are important ways to take care of our bodies and kill cancer cells or other immune suppressing disorders, beyond western medicine.

God Bless you all and more power to you in your fight against your cancer!

UPDATE

Rosie Fiercefighter Lindberg-Lakso

Hi Ladies,

I wanted to update my story. Last I wrote I was finishing my last rounds of Cisplatin and Etoposide. Well, I finished that and had a CT scan that revealed I was cancer-free on Oct. 27th, 2010. Two days later I started having some pain under my right arm that radiated through my chest and back. I thought I just pulled a muscle, but the pain was not getting better. So my doctors moved up my PET/CT scan to January 5th, 2011. This scan revealed that there was a tumor growing out of my fourth rib bone and my chest lymph nodes were growing too. I had a bone biopsy done and, sure enough, my Large Cell Neuroendocrine Carcinoma of the Cervix had spread, completely passing up my pelvic area and now residing in my chest. Which I think is interesting since Large Cell is usually a lung cancer, so no wonder it wants to be in my chest.

I went through three weeks of radiation treatments, which were very easy, and did the job. I no longer have pain and I don't feel the tumor growing out of my rib! Currently, I am undergoing more chemo with Taxol, to kill the rest of the cancer that's hanging out. Taxol has been a very easy chemo. I don't feel like a "cancer patient." I have good energy and a good appetite. I am able to take care of my kids, house and go to work.

This cancer is messing with the wrong person! I am a very strong person inside and out and I WILL beat this cancer! It will not defeat me!!! I am just fighting round #2.

I love you all and your strength and determination is only fueling my recovery.

Thank You,-Rosie

Allyson Strong

Hey all,

I'm 24 years old and my story began in September 2010. After some irregular bleeding, I went to my doctor and she attempted a PAP. There was too much bleeding so she said I would have to go to a different doctor for a colposcopy. When I had this done, the doctor told me there was definitely something wrong and I would need surgery, whether this was cancerous or not. We assumed then that it was cancer. The following week, she said what we had already believed to be true.

Within hours I had an appointment for the next week at Sloan-Kettering in NYC. After some testing, they found it to be at a stage IIB, and the surgeon recommended no surgery, but an aggressive combination of chemo/radiation. I quickly had my eggs frozen at NYU's fertility clinic and began treatment right away.

I had 28 days of external radiation, 4 internal radiations and 4 rounds of Etoposide/Cisplatin, with a few hospitalizations in between for dehydration and bad reactions. I finished treatment in early January.

I started to feel good again after a few weeks and was ready to get on with life, until I had my first scan on Feb 21st. We were completely floored on the 23rd, when we received the scans. There were 2 metastases to the liver and one, possibly very small one, on the lung. However, the tumor was gone from the cervix.

At this point my doctor said there was very little they could do except to try one more chemo, but think about quality of life.

This seemed absurd, and we refused to take that as an option. Since then, I have seen doctors at Columbia, Dana Farber and MD Anderson, as well as another specialist in NYC. All came up with the Taxol/Avastin route of chemotherapy and gave long-term and back-up options.

I will be getting a port next week, and will begin treatments with a Dr. Mitchell Gaynor. He also has put me on a large list of supplements to help with things ranging from the liver itself, to the side effects of treatments, to boosting the immune system to fighting the cancer. He also encourages meditation, visualizations and guided imagery.

Very close to Anderson was a park called Cancer Survivors Plaza. I took my picture in front of that plaque, because I know I will beat this. There was a beautiful fountain in the middle, and around the "walk" they posted inspiring plaques, which included my favorite:

"Realize that cancer is a life-threatening disease, but some beat it. Make up your mind you will be one of those who do."

Although they never got to write the end to their stories, I believe their words were left behind as a reminder to keep fighting.

These were strong, courageous and beautiful women. Their voices will be heard and their memories forever honored.

In Memoriam

Meredith Wright - 2007
Anne Childers - 2009
Shawna O'Brian - 2009
Morgan Jackson - 2009
Ally McLeod - 2010
Trudy Cooper - 2010
Sara Chalmers - 2010
Cristy Roberts - 2010
Sharon "Shaz" Thompson - 2010
Kristie Nelson - 2010
Amy Lynn - 2010
Michelle Planten - 2011
Cathryn Van Horn - 2012
Allyson Strong - 2011
Rosie Lindberg-Lakso – 2011
Candeese Dixon - 2011
Veronica Doyle-O'Meara – 2011

Meka Horne - 2011
Shawn Knutson – 2012
Marilyn Jackson – 2012
Kim Collins - 2012
Christinia Salinas - 2012
Crystal Jones - 2012
Honey Ji – 2012
Jamie Layton-Cagle - 2012
Jane McArthur - 2012
Jen Bell-Burgess - 2012
Katie Kalenze - 2012
Megan Byre - 2012
Meredith Gillespie - 2012
Sarah Molnar - 2012
Whitney Rybert – 2012
Carol Sissom - 2013
Pearlie Lance – 2013
Amber Korte – 2013
Meghan Capossere -2013
Becky Love – 2013
Lillian Kelly – 2013

The Sorority of Hope was written to tell the story of these amazing women who happen to be connected by one commonalty: this cancer diagnosis. The premise that started the movement was that no other women would ever feel alone and isolated in this diagnosis. We feel this goal has been achieved. Brining awareness to this disease so that people understand this isn't your garden variety cervical cancer, not all cervical cancer is caused by HPV, not all cervical cancer is 100% preventable and that this cancer will kill more than 80% of those diagnosed, is of the upmost importance, as is raising funds so that research may be done to find a protocol for effective treatment and someday, a cure. But what is most inspiring is the hope, love and strength that has brought these women together, to unite under one cause and reach out to each other in ways that no other circumstance could promote. The friendships brought together through this group will exist as positive energy longer than we will as humans.

Sorority of Hope will live on in the DNA of each of these women, who will strive to raise awareness and honor each other and those we have lost, through dignity, kindness and generosity.

Sorority of Hope

Afterward

In 2011, the first gathering of women diagnosed with this rare cancer took place in New York City, where 9 women surviving SCCC/LCCC and their supporters met for the first time. As you have read in this book, in 2012 a gathering took place in Las Vegas and I (Colleen Marlett) was fortunate to be able to attend. As described, it was a magical event, surpassing all expectations. I feel so lucky to have been able to meet the women I have, and form the bonds that we now share because of this terrible disease. Or is it something else that binds us?

In Vegas last year, I met a woman by the name of Pearlie Lance. I shared a room with her for 4 days, along with Melanie and Toni. It was my first time meeting Melanie in person, but because we had shared so much, it was like I'd just seen her the week before. Between Mel and I, one will start a sentence and the other will finish it. We are connected like the Pisces fish symbol we share, albeit Mel is usually the fish swimming with the tide and I the one swimming against it. With Pearlie it was different, yet much the same.

Pearlie emanates her faith from every fiber of her being. Her strength, hope and love are invulnerable. In her, I found acceptance to be who I am, without apology. She offered me friendship and, at times, tough love. She touched my soul in a way no one, ever in my life has been able to do. She gave me a place, for once, where I felt I belonged and showed me what true grit and valor are really all about. She is a woman of integrity, wit, wisdom and strength. With grace and dignity she offered me the gift of her friendship, which did not come easily for her with anyone. Although she is a woman of tolerance, she is no fool and could spot a hypocrite a mile away. I love that about her.

On January 11th, 2013 her journey took her home. I realize I speak of her as if she is still with us on earth because, for me, she always will be. For me this diagnosis, battle and all that this journey has entailed is worth every minute, for knowing Pearlie Lance. This year in Vegas, I lived and witnessed more of these life-changing experiences. I am looking forward to 2014

The word "sorority" is defined as: A group of girls or women associated for a common purpose; a sisterhood. Our purpose is Hope. We are women connected by possibility. We are the women of the "Sorority of Hope". We are "Rare but There"!

To find us on Facebook, please go to this link and ask to join our group. https://www.facebook.com/groups/scccsisters/

"If you bring forth what is within you, what you bring forth will save you. If you do not bring forth what is within you, what you do not bring forth will destroy you."

Jesus

Christ